Diode Lasers
in Neurosurgery

ISBN : 2-7420-0267-16

Éditions John Libbey Eurotext
127, avenue de la République
92120 Montrouge, France.
Tél. : 01 46 73 06 60
Site internet : http://www.john-libbey-eurotext.fr

John Libbey & Company Ltd
13, Smiths Yard, Summerley Street
London SW18 4HR
England.
Tel. : 1947 27 77

John Libbey CIC
Via L. Spallanzani, 11
00161, Roma, Italia.
Tel. : 06 862 289

© John Libbey Eurotext. Paris : 1999

Il est interdit de reproduire intégralement ou partiellement le présent ouvrage sans autorisation de l'éditeur ou du Centre Français d'Exploitation du Droit de Copie (CFC), 20, rue des Grands-Augustins, 75006 Paris.

Diode Lasers in Neurosurgery

François-Xavier Roux
Bertrand Devaux

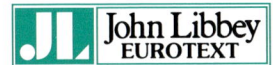

The publication of this book was made possible
thanks to DIOMED Limited, Cambridge, United Kingdom.

Contents

■ History of the use of lasers in neurosurgery . . 7

■ The physics of lasers 11

■ Types of laser 19

■ Physiological data 31

■ Lasers and safety 35

■ Technical data 41

■ Neurosurgical applications for diode lasers . 51

■ Future perspectives 75

■ Bibliography 79

■ References relevant to other types of surgery . . 83

■ Index 85

History of the use of lasers in neurosurgery

The discipline of neurosurgery was only born at the beginning of the 20th century, since which time a whole series of technical and technological advances have resulted in steadily improving clinical results. The first great step forward was the introduction by Harvey Cushing in 1926 of the technique of electrocoagulation for controlled haemostasis. Forty years later, Y. Yasargil (Zurich, Switzerland) and T. Kurze (Los Angeles, USA) developed, if not actually invented the technique of micro-neurosurgery, thus giving birth to modern neurosurgery. It was not until the end of the 1970's that laser technology first began to be applied to neurosurgery.

The theoretical bases of LASER (Light Amplification by Stimulated Emission of Radiation) radiation follow on from the work of Albert Einstein, specifically from the principles of energy quantization (Planck, 1900; Einstein, 1905) and the particle theory of electromagnetic radiation which holds that light is a form of particulate electromagnetic radiation in which the particles are called photons: each photon represents the fundamental amount (or "packet") of energy of a light particle or quantum which is equal to hν (where h is the Universal Planck constant and ν is the frequency of the radiation).

In 1917, Albert Einstein published papers on the absorption and emission of light in which the ideas of spontaneous and stimulated emission were proposed for the first time. In this revolutionary work, Einstein was already talking about stimulated emission: electromagnetic radiation would stimulate certain molecules or atoms to emit photons of energy hν, which photons would in turn be absorbed by other atoms or molecules leading to a chain reaction of stimulated emission and amplification of the light.

In 1954, on the basis of these early hypotheses, Townes developed the MASER (Microwave Amplification by Stimulated Emission of Radiation) and, together with Schawlow, demonstrated that it was theoretically possible to generate coherent light by inducing stimulated emission in an optical resonator.

In 1960 in the United States, Maiman developed the first laser oscillator with a gain medium consisting of a crystal of ruby and one year later, Javan and Bennet developed the first gas laser which was based on a mixture of Helium and Neon.

In 1964, Patel developed the CO_2 laser and, at around the same time, the first Argon and Neodymium-YAG lasers were constructed. In 1958, Bassov had proposed that a laser could be based on semiconducting materials and, in 1962, such machines were constructed more or less simultaneously in the laboratories of IBM, General Electric and the Massachusetts Institute of Technology (MIT). In 1964, three researchers – N.G. Bassov (USSR), C.H. Townes (USA) and A.M. Prokhorov (USSR) – were awarded the Nobel Prize for Physics for their joint contributions to the discovery of the Laser Effect. The parentage of the laser was truly international.

Following this period of purely scientific and technological progress, there came a period of animal experimentation which soon began to focus on the central nervous systems (K.M. Earle, S. Carpentier *et al.*, 1965; J.L. Fox, J.R. Hayes and M.N. Stein, 1965; T.E. Brown, C. True and R.L. McLaurin, 1966) of rats and dogs using either ruby or argon lasers. Early results were unimpressive but at least a new area of research had been opened up; the full potential of applying laser technology to neurosurgery did not become apparent until Stellar published the results of his experiments with CO_2 lasers in 1969 and 1974.

The current ways in which lasers – in this case CO_2 lasers – are used were really first developed in 1976-1977 by T. Takizawa in Japan, O.J. Beck in Germany and P.W. Ascher in Austria. The interest of North American, French and Italian neurosurgeons in laser applications only really began to take root as of the first conference on Lasers and Neurosurgery which took place in Chicago in 1981. These days, lasers are routine tools in many neurosurgery operating theatres but they should not be considered as a cure-all – they can only be accessory instruments of greater or lesser usefulness although they can be very effective and, in certain situations, irreplaceable. Without doubt, the use of lasers has vastly improved the efficiency with which certain tumours can be excised, *e.g.* those involving the posterior cranial fossa. In this respect, it parallels the technique of Cavitron UltraSound Aspiration (CUSA) with which it is often combined. These new options open up fascinating future possibilities, especially in terms of endoscopic applications, a subject to which we will return later on.

Two main different types of laser have been in regular use in neurosurgery over the last twenty years: the reference type remains the CO_2 laser, largely because its output radiation is efficiently absorbed by water molecules meaning that its penetration is limited in nervous tissue which has a relatively high water content (80%). Such instruments can be used for so-called "non-contact" applications with a highly focused beam to keep to a minimum any mechanical damage to local structures like the brain stem, the spinal cord and functionally important areas of the cortex. Such lasers are very effective at cutting and vaporising tumour and nervous tissue but less efficient at inducing haemostasis. The big disadvantage of CO_2 lasers is that their beam can only be directed via an articulated arm (at least for the time being) which significantly compromises their manoeuvrability and makes them unsuitable for endoscopy-type applications. Later, YAG lasers were applied to neurosurgery, largely because they present the advantage that their beam can be conducted through fibre optic making it more manoeuvrable and therefore more versatile. The resonator cavity of this type of laser is based on a crystal which contains three components, yttrium, aluminium and garnet. The YAG crystal emits in the infrared at a specific wavelength determined by the substance used to dope the crystal which is, in most cases, neodymium. A neodymium-YAG or Nd-YAG laser has a spectrum which includes over 20 different transitions between 939 and 1,440 nanometres (nm). The two most useful of these are at 1,064 nm (λ = 1.06 µm) and at 1,318 nm (λ = 1.32 µm). Alternatively, YAG crystals can be doped with other Rare Earth metals like erbium (λ = 2.9 µm) or holmium (λ = 2.1 µm); the holmium-YAG laser may well prove to be useful in neurosurgery in the future because its radiation, like that of a CO_2 laser, is efficiently absorbed by water molecules and hence by nervous tissue.

More recently, a novel type of machine has appeared which, in our opinion, represents a whole new generation of lasers which should see huge development in the coming years given the wide range of applications such machines are already being used for and the numerous potential applications being envisaged or currently under investigation: this is the **semiconductor diode laser**, the subject of this book.

The physics of lasers

■ Properties of light

Light is a form of energy which travels very fast (300,000 km/s) and which does not need a material substrate for its propagation since it can be transmitted through a vacuum. It can travel through the type of solid object which we call "transparent", which actually means that it does not absorb light to any great extent. Certain of the properties of light can only be explained if it is treated as a wave (*e.g.* diffraction and interference) whereas others can only be understood if it is considered as a particle (*e.g.* the photoelectric effect and stimulated emission). It was the French physicist Louis de Broglie who, combining the principles of the electromagnetic and wave radiation theory with those of quantum optics (photon radiation), discovered the relationship between the energy (E) of any particle and the frequency of its associated wave form (ν) such that $E = h\nu$, where h is a universal constant (the Planck's constant) equal to $6.6252.10^{-34}$ joule/s.

Therefore, light rays can be considered as streams of photons (electromagnetic, corpuscular or photon radiation) with each different type of light (or "colour") corresponding to a specific wavelength. The visible range of the electromagnetic spectrum is between $\lambda = 775$ nm (red light) and 375 nm (violet light). Beyond the red end of the spectrum lie infrared (IR) and then radio waves; beyond the other end of the visible spectrum lie ultraviolet (UV) rays, then X-rays, γ-rays and, with the shortest wavelengths, cosmic rays *(figure 1)*.

Normal light such as sunlight or that coming from a light bulb is a mixture of many different waves of different wavelengths which are out of phase with respect to one another. This type of light is also **scattered** in all directions so the energy of the photons is dissipated in the surrounding space. Such light or radiation is described as **incoherent and non monochromatic** *(figure 2)*.

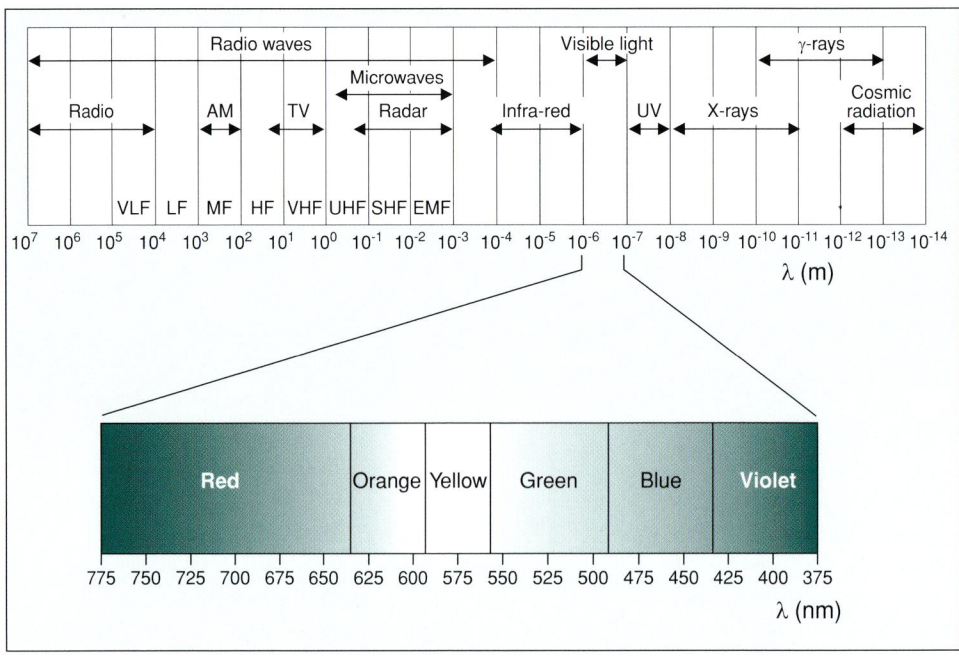

■ **Figure 1.** *The electromagnetic spectrum.*

In contrast, laser light is **coherent, monochromatic** and not subject to **scattering**. All the component waves remain in phase and each different laser radiation has its own specific colour depending on its specific wavelength: *e.g.* a Helium-Neon laser emits a red beam with a wavelength of 632.8 nm, an Argon laser emits either

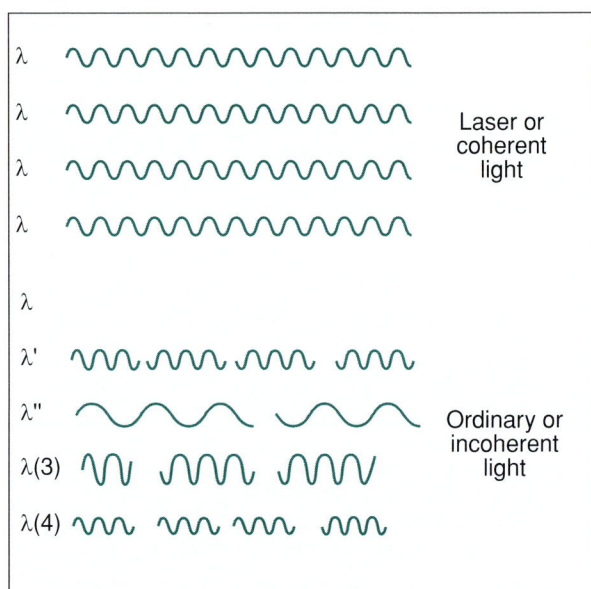

■ **Figure 2.** *A comparison of laser light (coherent) with normal light (incoherent).*

in the blue range (488 nm) or the green (514.5 nm), and CO_2 lasers emit in the infrared (10.6 µm). The kind of diode laser currently used for surgical applications like those used in neurosurgery also emit in the infrared range, usually at wavelengths of between 805 nm and 1,000 nm (= 1 µm). We are now going to outline how laser light is generated. The principal properties of this kind of radiation can be explained by reviewing the physical principles which govern the construction of a laser.

■ Spontaneous emission

In simplified terms, an atom consists of a nucleus around which electrons orbit. The paths or orbits of these electrons are associated with different energy levels and when an electron absorbs energy (*e.g.* electrical or in the form of light), it can jump from its current orbit to one associated with a higher energy which is further away from the nucleus. To change orbits in this way and pass into an "excited" state, the electron must absorb a quantum of energy $E = h\nu$. The lifetime of an excited electron is extremely short (10^{-8} s) meaning that it returns to its initial energy level, its original orbit, rapidly. When the electron returns to its original orbit, the energy stored during excitation has to be released and this occurs by means of the emission of a quantum of energy ($h\nu$) in the form of a photon. Since the return of the electron to its initial state is spontaneous, this kind of radiation is called "spontaneous emission". The frequency of the photon (ν) is directly proportional to the energy (E) which the electron originally absorbed to jump from an orbit with energy Ea to an orbit of higher energy level Eb *(figure 3)*.

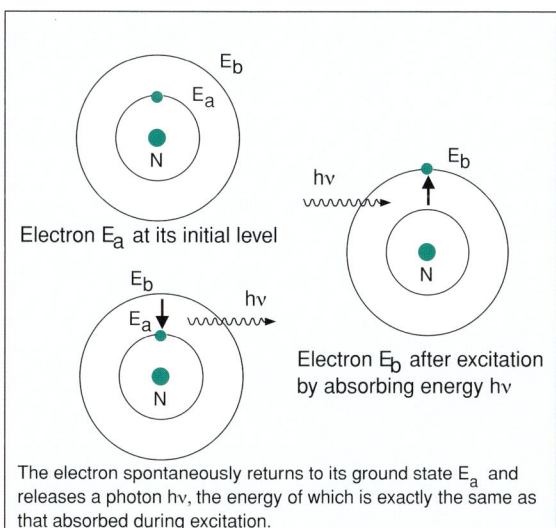

■ **Figure 3.** *The basis of spontaneous emission.*

Stimulated or induced emission

Where laser light is concerned, instead of waiting for the electron to fall back down to its initial level Ea spontaneously, the return is predicted and induced. Such "stimulated" or "induced" emission is obtained by using light radiation with exactly the same frequency (ν) and therefore the same energy (since E = hν) as that stored in the excited electron. Now the electron, in falling back down to its original energy level Ea, is going to emit two photons of exactly the same energy (hν), in one case the energy necessary to jump from orbit Ea to the next higher orbit Eb and, in the other case, the energy (hν) which induced the early return to the initial level of energy Ea. Not only does the second or "induced" photon have exactly the same energy as the first, but also all their other characteristics are the same including direction and polarisation. This process is cumulative because these last two photons go on to induce two more photons. Actually, the two emitted photons hν, in the course of their path through the excited material, meet other excited electrons. Thus, a whole series of photons with always the same frequency and energy hν are generated. The resultant stimulated emission is highly directional, very intense and perfectly uniform with respect to frequency and therefore wavelength λ. It is these characteristics which give laser radiation its special properties. The chain reaction proceeds and a beam of photons is generated, *i.e.* a beam of electromagnetic radiation in which all the photons have exactly the same frequency. Of course, this is a highly simplified description of an enormously complex phenomenon: in fact, there are not

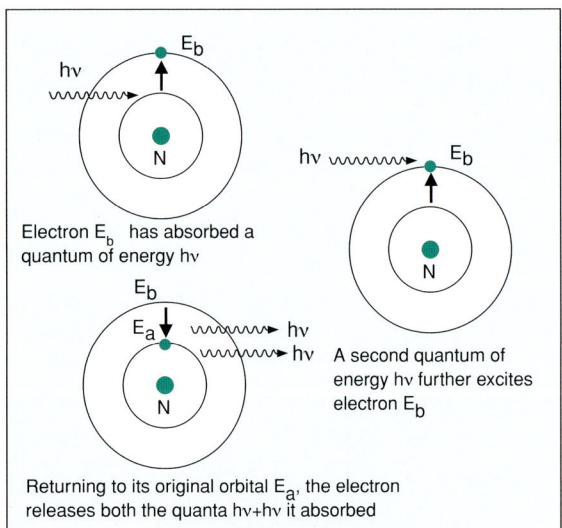

■ **Figure 4.** *The basis of stimulated emission.*

just two different energy levels but rather many and passage from a higher level down to a lower one can occur *via* several different steps, some spontaneous and some stimulated. In addition, the same kind of phenomenon can be applied not only to atoms but also to ions and molecules *(figure 4)*.

■ Laser emission

■ Necessary components *(figure 5)*

In order to generate a laser beam, the following are absolutely required:

1. **A gain medium** which can be excited and stimulated to release photons with the same frequency and energy. This medium is the heart of the laser and it might be a solid (a ruby or a YAG crystal), a gas (Helium-Neon, Argon or carbon dioxide) or a liquid (an organic dye). A diode can be used, *e.g.* a Ga As Al diode (aluminium-doped gallium arsenide).

2. **An energy pump** which is a system to excite usually electrically the atoms and molecules in the gain medium to maintain stimulated emission. In a laser, *"population inversion"* has to be maintained which means that the number of atoms excited up to energy level Eb must be greater than the number occupying the initial level Ea. Therefore, stimulated emission must predominate over absorption and this

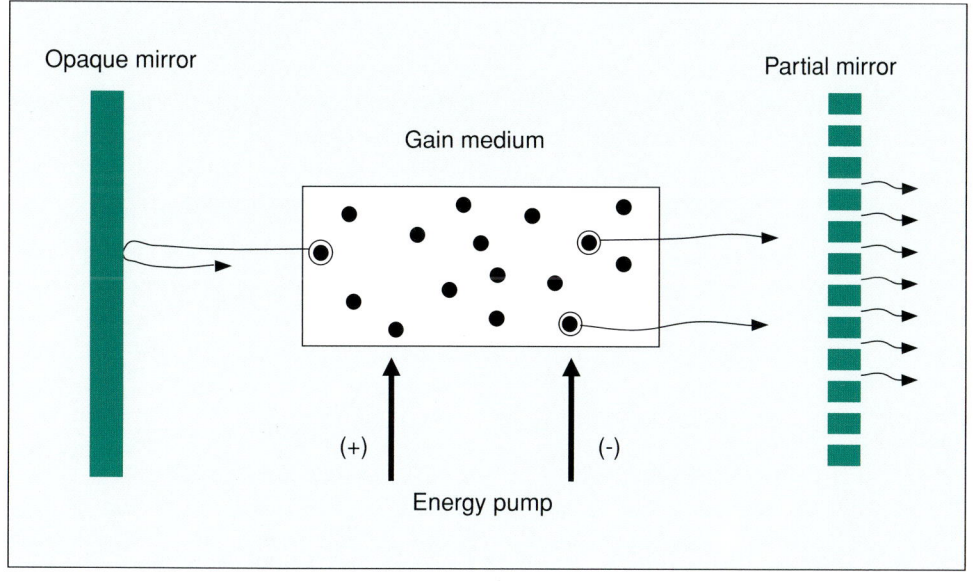

■ **Figure 5.** *The essential components in a laser device.*

requires rapid, efficient energy input into the gain medium – this is referred to as "pumping" and if the energy source is light, the term *"optical pumping"* is used. Optical pumping can be based on a conventional, incoherent light source like a flash or arc lamp or the source can be coherent, in which case a primary laser is used to pump the gain medium of the main laser, *e.g.* a diode laser can be used to pump a solid-state YAG laser. Other electronic pumping systems can also be used, based on electrical discharges or electron beams.

3. **A laser cavity** containing the gain medium and serving as a generator. Together, the gain medium and the pumping system can amplify but not generate light. To act as a generator, the amplifier has to be converted into an oscillator, *i.e.* some of the output photons have to be sent back into the amplifier *via* a mirror system. One of the mirrors must reflect all photons and is referred to as the "resonator"; the other is semi-transparent so it reflects some of the photons while at the same time allowing emission of the beam from the machine.

Coherent, monochromatic, directional

In contrast to incandescent lamps which emit spontaneously and generate incoherent beams of photons, lasers emit coherent beams with a specific wavelength. By means of the mechanism described above, all components of the laser beam are in perfect phase with one another and therefore interfere positively. This means that in a laser all waves vibrate similarly and in phase. These laser phases feature a high degree of correlation both in space – any two points on a given perpendicular section are in phase **(spatial coherence)** – and in time – the same phase difference is maintained between any two different instants at the same point in space **(temporal coherence)**. It is this high degree of coherence which makes laser beams thoroughly **directional** and **monochromatic**, the two characteristics which distinguish this form of radiation.

• **Monochromatic** means that the radiated beam has a very narrow bandwidth, a property which is due to the fact that the intra-atomic or intra-molecular electronic transitions from which it results are very tightly defined. This is almost synonymous with coherence. A monochromatic beam, then, is one with a very small bandwidth which either does not diverge at all or diverges very little.

• **Directional** means that the laser beam can be accurately pointed and used for surgical applications. The beam only diverges by a matter of a few thousandths of a radian because the resonator cavity mirror system allows out only those photons travelling in a certain direction. This results in a beam of light, the power of which is highly concentrated in space. Radiation from an incoherent light source is omnidirectional whereas a laser emits an almost perfectly parallel beam of light. For illustration, a typical degree of divergence might result in a laser illuminating a circle of just one meter in diameter at a point one kilometre distant from the source – the corresponding surface which would be illuminated by an incoherent light source of the same energy output would be 16 million times greater. By way of further illustration, the luminance in the red range of a simple helium-neon laser which is emitting a few kilowatts of light energy is one thousand times greater than that of the Sun. Finally, by means of relatively unsophisticated focusing systems based on optical elements like mirrors and lenses, beams with intensities that could not have been envisaged even a few years ago are now easy to generate, *e.g.* intensities of up to 1,020 watts per square centimetre (W/cm^2) are attainable with lasers emitting extremely short pulses in the femtosecond range (1 fs = 10^{-15} s).

■ Laser beam energy parameters

■ Emission power

The power output of a laser can be measured with either a Wattmeter or a Joulemeter which is suitable for the type of laser concerned. A power of 1 watt corresponds to an emitted energy of 1 Joule per second:

$$1 \text{ W} = 1 \text{ J} \times 1 \text{ s.}$$

The instantaneous power P(t) being emitted by a laser at a given instant t is given by P(t) = dE / dt, where dE is the amount of energy (in Joules) emitted between the two time points t and t + dt (in seconds).

When a laser is being operated continuously, P(t) remains constant over time but, when it is being operated in modulated or pulsed mode, P(t) fluctuates with time.

■ Irradiance and power density

Irradiance I is the amount of power delivered per unit area. The mean irradiance over a specific surface is given by:

$$I_{mean} = P(t) / \text{total surface area}$$

and local irradiance by:

$$I_{local} = dP / dS$$

(dP = instantaneous power delivered to an element with an area of dS).

The SI unit for irradiance is Watts per square meter (W/m²) but, in practice, units of W/cm² or W/mm² are more common.

Because of its special properties, notably its coherence, laser light disperses to a very small extent and therefore loses energy very slowly. Moreover, if it is focused using a lens or some other kind of optical system, its energy can be concentrated into a very tiny area – it is this property which makes it so useful in surgery. The diameter of the beam at the point of focus can theoretically be reduced to the same order of magnitude as the wavelength of the laser light concerned thus making it possible to deliver very high densities of power and energy. Thus, the beam from a small laser (1 mW) focused to a point of 1 µm in diameter would give a power density of 100 kW/cm² – the sun delivers about 0.1 kW/cm². Power Density (PD) is directly proportional to emission power and inversely proportional to the targeted surface area (St):

$$PD = Pe / St$$

where:
– PD = power density (expressed in W/mm²)
– Pe = emission power (in W)
– St = targeted surface area (in mm²).

Since the area covered by the beam is proportional to the square of its diameter ($S = \pi d^2/4$), for every doubling of the diameter of the beam at the point of impact, the power density is reduced by a factor of four. Therefore, by adjusting the focusing of the beam, it is possible to modulate its effect on the target area – we will come back to this useful practical option in chapter 7 (see "Operating procedure").

Types of laser

This book is mainly concerned with semiconductor diode lasers but it seems worthwhile nevertheless to mention certain other types of machine in order to provide the reader with as much information as possible on the different kinds of laser source which are currently being used in neurosurgery.

■ Carbon dioxide lasers

As mentioned above, **CO_2 lasers** are the reference instruments for surgery involving the central nervous system. In practice, the actual gas used is a mixture which only contains 6% carbon dioxide together with 20% nitrogen and 74% helium. Such machines emit in the infrared so the beam is invisible – for this reason, a cold (with an emission power of between 0.1 and 1 mW), "tracer" beam of visible, red light ($\lambda = 0.6328$ µm) generated with a helium-neon laser is superimposed on the active beam for visualisation purposes.

The main advantage of this kind of laser light is that, with a wavelength of 10.6 µm *(see figure 6)*, it is efficiently absorbed by water molecules which represent the main constituent of nervous tissue. The result of its being efficiently absorbed is that it does not penetrate into the underlying, deep cerebral tissue. This kind of laser can be used for non-contact applications and is easy to focus. CO_2 lasers are very effective at cutting and vaporising tumour and nervous tissue but less good for inducing haemostasis. The big disadvantage of CO_2 lasers is that their beam can only be directed *via* an articulated arm which significantly compromises their manoeuvrability and makes them unsuitable for either neuroendoscopy-type applications or for minimally invasive, stereotactically guided procedures. We have been using a CO_2 laser for many years because, as is the case for anyone who has been exploiting this technology since the early 1980's, this was the only type of laser source available.

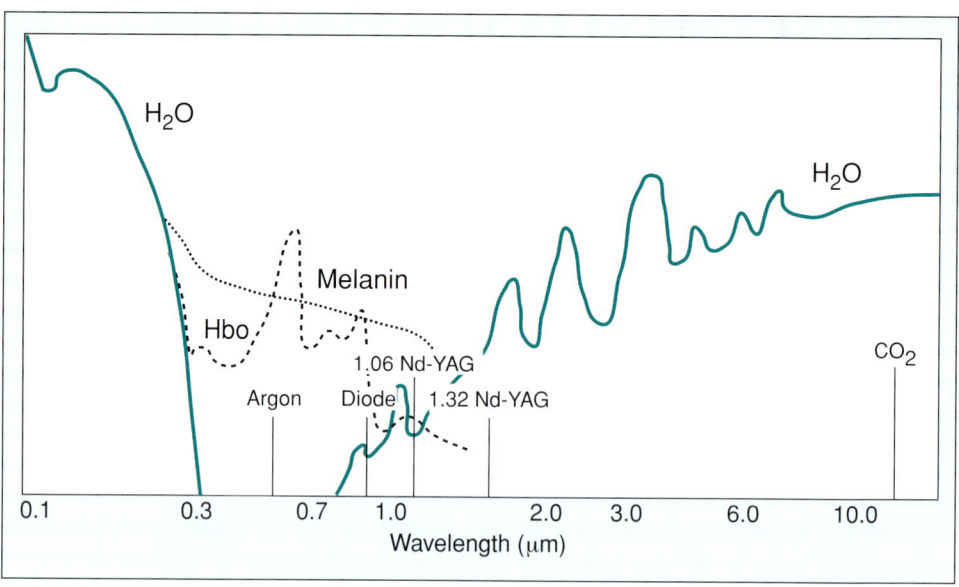

Figure 6. *Absorption by water and important chromophores at different wavelengths.*

In the next chapter, we will deal with the effects of CO_2 and various other types of laser (including Nd-YAG and semiconductor models) as revealed by histology of the brains of experimentally treated rats and rabbits.

The components of a CO_2 laser

The housing contains the generator and its accessories. The control panel includes, as for any surgical laser unit, controls for adjusting emission power, setting exposure times and selecting either continuous, pulsed or superpulsed operation mode.

The power delivered varies from one model to another and from one manufacturer to another but is usually up to somewhere between 20 and 100 W in continuous mode emission (cw) and up to 300-400 W in pulsed mode. In today's neurosurgical procedures, high powers are not needed and a maximum emission power of between 20 and 25 W is nearly always more than enough.

Unfortunately, **an articulated arm** is necessary to conduct the infrared beam of a CO_2 laser to the hand piece. This arm usually takes the form of two rigid but fairly light tubes with six or seven joints. Each joint is made up of two different elements, each of which can be turned through an angle of 360° with respect to the other. Inside the joints are mirrors inclined at angles of 45° such that the beam is reflected through a total angle of 90° in the plane of incidence of the mirror. The hand piece is equipped with a joint system containing seven mirrors by means of which the beam can be sent in any direction required in the operating zone. The articulated arm is an extremely delicate device which is very sensitive to shock, vibrations and mechanical perturbation, all of which can easily disturb the finely balanced optical system and throw off course either the CO_2 beam or the helium-neon tracer. Another disadvantage of this arm system is that it significantly restricts manoeuvrability, which precludes endoscopy-type applications for this class of laser.

On the other hand, a micromanipulator can be fitted to the end of the articulated arm to allow it to be used in conjunction with an operating microscope. With this device, the beam can be moved without adjusting the focus of the microscope, and the focus of the beam itself can be adjusted according to whether it is being used for cutting or coagulation. In practice, we have not actually used the micromanipulator very extensively because it still further cuts down on both the operator's ability to direct the beam and its manoeuvrability – we have usually chosen to use the hand piece on its own.

The hand piece contains two main components, a body which contains the lenses (50, 125 or 200 mm) used for focusing the beam and an adapter at the distal end where mirrors can be installed at an oblique angle to turn the beam through either 45° or 60° – this system somewhat enhances the manoeuvrability of the hand piece. Some hand pieces are also fitted with a device to change the focal point of the beam (a "zoom" type optical system) in order to vary its diameter at the impact point between 0.3 and 3 mm.

Accessories are available for CO_2 lasers which offer improved manoeuvrability over conventional hand pieces (but never as good manoeuvrability as that of fibre optic-based systems): these are called *wave guides*. Hollow wave guides are semi-rigid ceramic tubes in which the beam is propagated in more or less the same way as it is in fibre optic. These devices are made to be fitted to the optical arm outlet but the resultant beam is divergent so if a focused beam is needed, yet another optical element is necessary. These accessories have never been shown to be very useful, at least not in neurosurgery.

A number of investigations into the possibility of conducting CO_2 laser beams through fibre optic have been undertaken in recent years but it has not yet been shown that the flexibility and transmission efficiency of such systems is adequate for surgical applications.

Solid-state lasers: YAG lasers

YAG laser beams have the advantage that they are transmitted *via* fibre optic which makes them manoeuvrable and suitable for certain specific types of procedure involved in cerebral surgery including endoscopy. In addition, the hand pieces which do not have to contain any kind of mirrors or special optical devices are far smaller and lighter than those associated with CO_2 lasers. This means that deep lesions can be removed through limited approaches such as those performed in stereotactically guided procedures.

In this type of laser, the resonator cavity is based on a crystal containing three components, yttrium, aluminium and garnet. The specific wavelength emitted by this crystal depends on the doping substance used, which can be one of a variety of trivalent Rare Earth metal ions but is usually neodymium (Nd^{3+}), to give a neodymium-YAG or Nd-YAG laser which has a spectrum with over 20 different transitions between 939 and 1,440 nm: the two most useful of these for medical applications are at 1.06 µm (1,064 nm) and 1.32 µm (1,318 nm). Alternatively, the YAG crystal can be doped with other Rare Earth metals like erbium (Er-YAG, λ = 2.9 µm) or holmium (Ho-YAG, λ = 2.1 µm).

Nd-YAG lasers can be used in two different ways:
1. continuous emission for conventional or stereotactically guided surgery and endoscopy;
2. short pulse emission (triggered) – this mode is only ever used in ophthalmology, specifically in the correction of cataract.

In the first case, a rod of about ten centimetres in length and 8 millimetres in diameter is optically pumped by a pair of DC krypton lamps to give laser powers of the order of 100 W at the tip of the fibre. In the second example, the rod is 5 centimetres long and 3 millimetres in diameter and is excited by a small linear xenon flash lamp which emits a few Joules within a time frame of about 50 microseconds – this gives several milliJoules of laser energy concentrated into a few nanoseconds, enough to perform ocular capsulotomy.

In neurosurgery, the future value of YAG lasers may depend on the versatility due to the fact that they can emit at two different wavelengths, 1.06 and 1.32 µm. The first wavelength can also be doubled in frequency using a KTP (potassium, Titanyl, phosphate) crystal to emit in the green range (λ = 532 nm), which beam can then be used in turn to pump a tunable dye laser to give another range of wavelengths in the red (λ = 0.62 µm; 0.67 µm) for the photochemotherapeutic treatment of cancer masses. This last application is still in the research stage and is therefore not relevant to current neurosurgical practice.

It seems important to highlight the fact that **the future of Nd-YAG lasers** depends on their potential for miniaturisation. This could be achieved by using **semiconductor diode lasers for optical pumping** which would also massively improve overall efficiency from 1% to 10%.

Dye lasers

Insofar as photochemotherapy has no current clinical applications in neurosurgery, we will just mention the existence of dye lasers, the use of which is restricted to photochemotherapeutic applications (or photodynamic therapy = PDT).

Diode lasers

Definition of a light-emitting diode

A semiconductor diode is an electronic component which emits light when an electric current is passed through it.

Light-emitting diodes (LED's) are the most common light source in electronic equipment, *e.g.* they are widely used in devices for displaying the time or other types of data on screens. With a few minor differences, a semiconductor laser functions in much the same way as a LED but emits far more powerful radiation. The main application for diode lasers is to run telecommunications fibre optic systems and their applications in medicine and surgery are significantly less economically important.

The basic configuration of a semiconductor diode laser is essentially the same as that of a LED, *i.e.* a positive-negative (p-n) junction with the only difference being the direction of the potential difference. The p-n junction is composed of a layer of synthetic crystal which is doped with atoms with a valence lower than that of the crystal material (p-type semiconductor) interfacing with another layer of the same crystal doped with atoms with a higher valence (n-type semiconductor). A migration current creates an electric field directed towards the p pole. In a LED, a potential difference is applied across the diode which prevents current passing in the absence of light.

In a semiconductor diode laser, light is generated by stimulated rather than by spontaneous emission which means that it can generate higher energy levels than a LED.

■ How semiconductor diode lasers work

Therefore, as just described, in semiconductor (diode) lasers, the junction between two different semiconducting materials constitutes the gain medium (the resonator cavity). The active layer comprises a 0.1 to 0.3 µm-thick layer of an aluminium-doped crystal of gallium arsenide (Ga Al As) sandwiched between two other layers (constituting a "double heterojunction"), on one side a layer of Ga As and on the other side a layer of Ga Al As with the one representing the negative pole n and the other the positive p *(figure 7)*. When a current passes across this junction, stimulated emission (the laser effect) occurs. To pump the diode, an electric current is applied between two layers of metal which function as electrodes arranged as a comb, *i.e.* in a network. The whole unit is very small, no larger than a few hundred microns

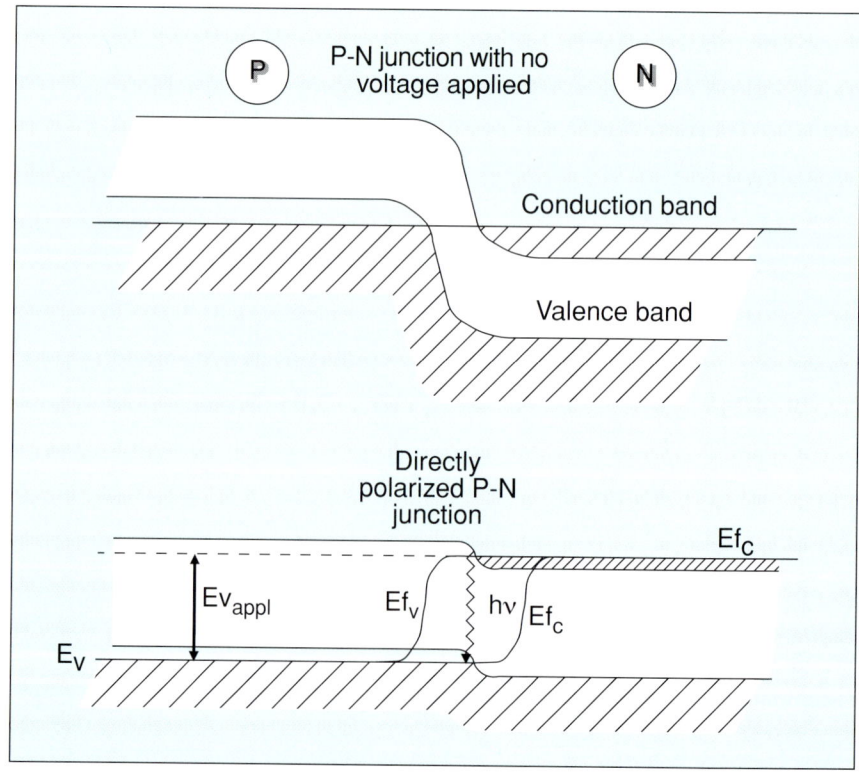

■ **Figure 7.** *A diagram of different energy levels in a semiconductor diode.*

(500 × 500 × 100 µm) *(figure 8)*. The efficiency of the conversion of electrical energy into light energy is relatively high – of the order of between 30% and 50%. Most of these lasers emit in the near infrared, between 800 and 900 nm but other wavelengths can be generated by using other semiconducting materials as the active crystal. The resultant beam is conical and very divergent (by a factor of between 15° to 30°) and therefore needs to be focused to give a good beam shape. Each optoelectronic chip emits a relatively low-power output (from a few tens of milliwatts to second generation chips of 2 W or 4 W output) but large numbers of individual units can be integrated to create arrays or matrices which generate laser beams of sufficient power for surgical use as is the case for any powerful laser. Thus surgical diode lasers can be constructed with power outputs of up to 60 W.

Such lasers have two main applications:
1. to pump another laser, *e.g.* as already mentioned, YAG lasers are often pumped with a diode laser;
2. for surgery, in the true sense, as will be described in chapters 6 and 7.

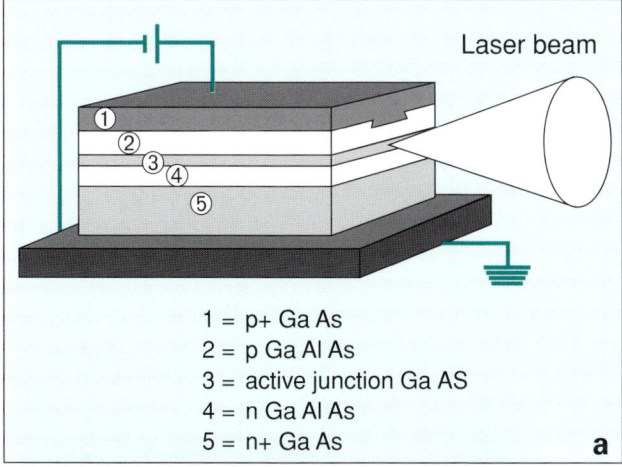

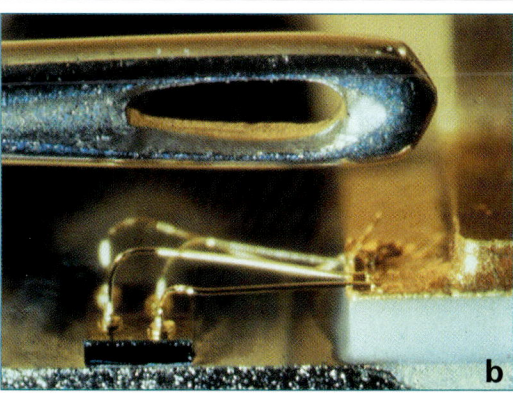

■ **Figure 8.** *The heterojunction diode laser.*
a) Diagrammatic representation. b) Micrograph of a 2 W diode showing its size relative to a needle's eye.

Transmission of semiconductor diode laser beams

As mentioned above, diode lasers emit in the near infrared range of the spectrum ($\lambda = 810 \pm 25$ nm). The resultant output beam is then sent along special optical fibres ("fibre optic") which efficiently conduct light in the near ultraviolet ($\lambda = 0.4$ µm) and near infrared ($\lambda = 1.5$ µm) ranges of the spectrum. Fibre optic is very fine and flexible so it is ideal for directing laser beams for endoscopically or microscopically controlled minimally invasive surgical procedures guided by stereotactic techniques or interventional navigation systems.

Light rays can be transmitted down a fibre *(figure 9a and b)* by virtue of two physical phenomena, *i.e.* that of total reflection at the interface between two dielectric media, and that of curvature of the path of the ray. The ray is propagating in a non-homogenous medium (doped silica) which is covered by a cylindrical outer layer made of a homogenous dielectric material (quartz fibres). These two different media – the core and the sheath – each have different light propagation indices with that of the sheath being lower than that of the core. Within the core, the propagation index decreases in a linear fashion as one moves from the centre out to the periphery towards the core-sheath interface. Finally, the whole assembly is covered in a protective coating. Light rays travelling through the core undergo total reflection at the core-sheath interface and therefore propagate all the way down the fibre without any attenuation assuming that both core and sheath materials are perfectly transparent.

Mounting the fibre on the laser source is obviously a problem insofar as the beam coming out of the laser cavity (*i.e.* the semiconductor laser array) has to be matched to and channelled down the core of the fibre in which it is to propagate. In practice, the fibre is moun-

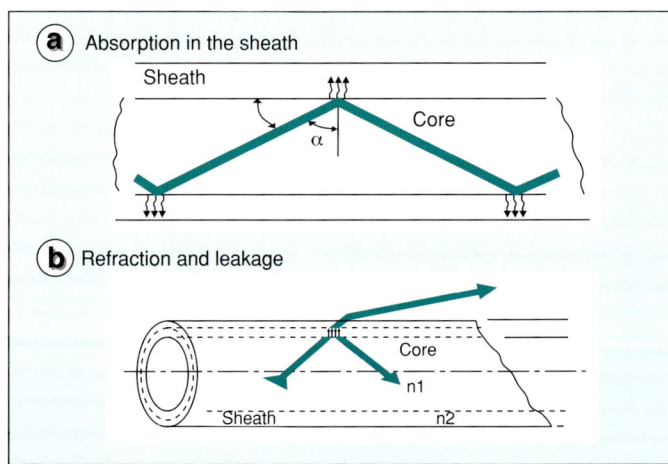

■ **Figure 9.** *Propagation of a laser beam down a fibre optic. a) Absorption by the sheath. b) Refraction and a leakage ray.*

ted on a micrometer system which can be adjusted to perfectly align the direction of the fibre with that of the laser beam and then centre the latter on the core of the fibre. Sometimes faulty alignment can lead to problems of imperfect beam transmission; therefore it is always essential to check that the mounting ring is correctly positioned as soon as the laser is turned on and whenever beam transmission seems to be falling off or power seems to be low in the course of an actual surgical procedure.

Two different phenomena can lead to the beam being transported down the fibre **losing energy**. Firstly, a small amount of energy is in fact *absorbed* by the sheath material every time the beam is reflected at the core-sheath interface so the more often the beam is reflected, the greater the amount of energy will be lost, attenuation which can become significant if the fibre is long and tortuous. Absorption in the fibre creates overheating which can lead to the melting of the protective coating and the fibre itself. This is the case mainly with high-power infrared lasers. This is usually only a problem when high-power infrared lasers are being used with highly absorbent fibres without any cooling system, such as high power diode lasers. The other phenomenon which can cause loss of energy from a laser beam is *diffusion*, which is associated with the existence of microscopic local variations in refractive index in the core material. In fact, it is considered that the centre of diffusion of the fibre becomes excited by the laser radiation and re-emits a fraction of the light energy so that refracted and leakage rays are generated at this centre of diffusion. This is why some of the energy is lost before it reaches the tip of the fibre. It should be noted that, for a given fibre, such diffusion phenomena become more significant as the wavelength of the radiation approaches the ultraviolet, as in excimer lasers. Therefore, for diode lasers which emit at the other end of the visible electromagnetic spectrum in the infrared range, losses due to diffusion phenomena are relatively small. On the other hand, peroperative manipulations can give rise to energy losses because of the constant bending and twisting of the fibre which abolishes the guided rays – wherever the fibre is curved, the only rays which propagate are the refracted or leakage rays which cause significant energy losses. This can be clearly seen by inspecting a fibre with a transparent protective coating being used with a helium-neon laser which emits a red beam: when the fibre is curved, the curved part can be seen to become illuminated as a result of the light leaking out of the core of the fibre and diffusing within the covering. This leakage is the reason why excessive bending of laser fibres should be avoided and why such fibres should generally be subjected to as little mechanical stress as possible.

When using a laser fibre, it is important to know or ascertain the parameters and the profile of the energy coming out of the tip of the fibre. There are two types of energy profile. The first type is *radial distribution* as observed where the beam is coming out from the transversely sectioned end of the fibre *(the near field)*. The second type is *angular distribution* which is how the energy profile of the ray appears after it has travelled a few centimetres from this same exit point *(the far field)*. Depending on the type of procedure being carried out, lasers are used in either contact or non-contact mode which is to say that the laser energy is delivered either with the fibre in direct contact with the tissue or only after focusing the output with a lens to generate a convergent or pseudo-parallel beam. Without going into all the details, it is enough to know that the distribution characteristics of these forms of laser energy can be calculated on the basis of the simple principles of geometrical optics (as long as it can be safely assumed that the fibre is rectilinear and non-diffusing). The approximations involved are justified as long as the fibre is short enough, as is the case in medical and surgical applications where the fibres are of the order of 3 to 4 meters in length. Thus, if the fibre core is being excited by a laser beam correctly aligned in the direction of the fibre, the transverse distribution of the ray in the far field takes the form of a cone whereas in the near field, it is more or less uniform *(figure 10)*.

Sapphires are optical elements which can be mounted directly at the tip of a laser fibre to focus the beam. The focusing occurs so close to the sapphire that it can be considered as occurring actually at its surface with next to no loss of energy through diffusion. There exists a variety of different sized and shaped sapphires which can be used to adapt the laser for use in contact mode for either sectioning tissue or inducing coagulation *(figure 11)* without generating any smoke or only very little.

Shaped fibres are a relatively recent technological development. The quartz tip of the fibre is moulded into shapes similar to those of the sapphires just discussed so that a shaped fibre could be said to have a sapphire element already built in. The advantages of this are considerable in that, not only are costs reduced but also energy losses and water or air cooling requirements associated with the fibre-sapphire interface are avoided. Moreover, the focusing of the laser beam in a shaped fibre, just like in a sapphire, occurs so close to the impact point that it can be considered that it actually really is occurring at the surface of the tip. For our work, we have not used sapphires for our beams for some years now – **we always use shaped quartz fibres**.

Types of laser

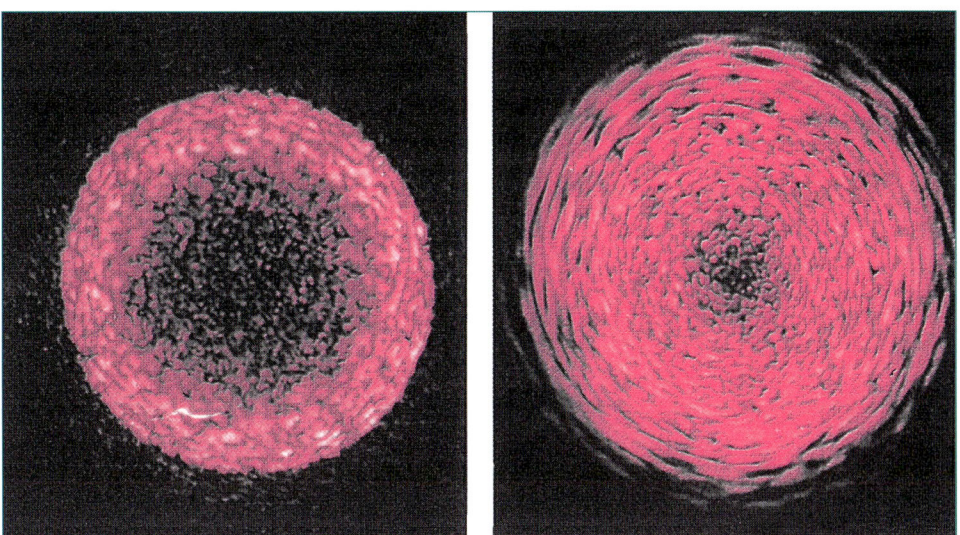

Figure 10. *Profile of rays in the near field (right) and the far field (left).*

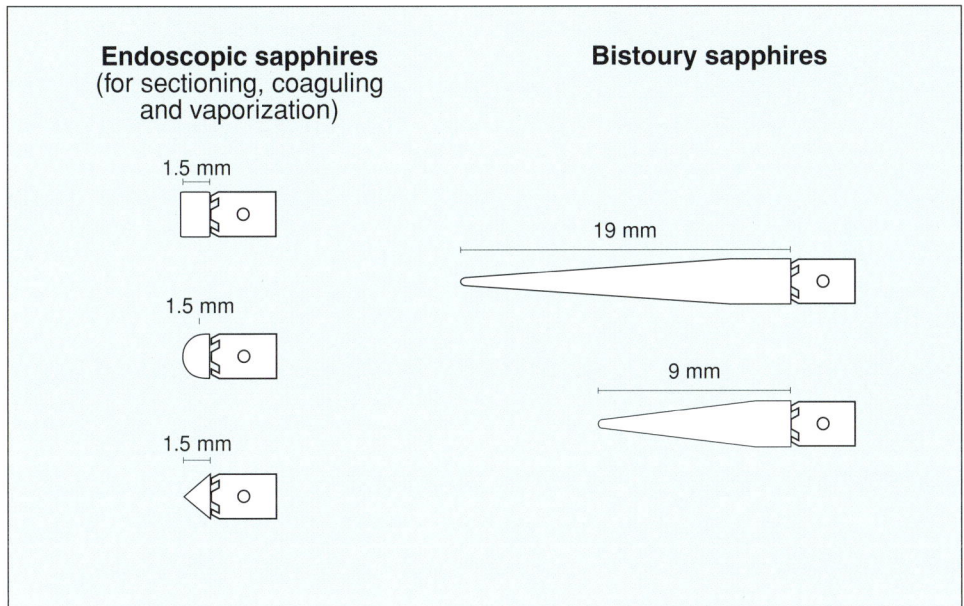

Figure 11. *Various shapes of sapphires used for endoscopic or free-hand procedures.*

There are two main types of shaped fibre:

1. the conical type has a tip measuring 300 µm – this type is suitable for making very fine incisions and sections with effective haemostasis and a minimum of damage to the tissue with which it is in contact;

29

2. spherical-type shaped fibres have diameters of either 800, 1,200 or 3,000 µm and are suitable for less fine work, either sectioning, vaporising or haemostasis, especially the last.

The disadvantage of shaped fibres is that care must be applied in their use as they are relatively delicate and sensitive to high temperatures at which they may well melt. These fibres are not actively cooled by water or air. In use the heat generated by the laser energy is conducted into the tissue itself. Therefore with excessive laser power, the tissue is unable to absorb all the heat generated. For these reasons, they should only be used with continuously operating lasers with a power output of 10 W or less. In general, for neurosurgical procedures, we use an output power of between 4 and 10 W cw with shaped fibres whatever the diameter (600 or 1,000 µm).

Physiological data

The exact physiological effects of lasers are primarily related to the mode of operation, *i.e.* cw or pulsed. The way in which a laser pulse interacts with a target biological tissue depends on several different parameters:
– firstly, the **irradiance** (the peak density of the power delivered per unit area, expressed in W/cm^2);
– secondly, the **interaction time** (in s);
– and thirdly, the **fluence** (or energy delivered per unit area, expressed in J/cm^2).

In practice, continuous or quasi-continuous lasers can be considered as mainly acting *via* thermal and photochemical mechanisms whereas pulsed lasers induce mainly electromechanical effects and photoablation. Electromechanical effects are induced with lasers emitting extremely short pulses, anything from a few tens picoseconds (1 ps = 10^{-12} s) to a few hundred nanoseconds (1 ns = 10^{-9} s).

Since diode lasers are exclusively used in surgery to induce thermal effects, in this chapter we will only deal with thermal aspects of laser-tissue interactions.

■ Laser-tissue interactions: general data

The extent of thermally induced tissue damage depends on the actual temperature reached and the time for which the concerned tissue was maintained at a temperature above the critical coagulation threshold. Any prolonged delivery of laser energy shot induces a local increase in temperature and the resultant tissue damage is due to the transfer of heat, the characteristics of which are dependent on the thermal properties of the specific tissue. In addition, the creation of a focal heat source depends on the optical properties of the tissue concerned. However, as the temperature increases, the optical and thermal properties of the tissue change together with changes in many of the other physicochemical properties of the local tissue. For this reason, in non-contact mode, rather than long, low-power exposures, repeated, short (between 1 and 30 ms) high-power pulses are preferable because during the interval period after each pulse, any heat generated by deposition of the laser energy has the time to dissipate in the surrounding tissue without the temperature steadily continuing to increase to very high levels.

The morphological changes induced and the extent of the denaturation of target tissues depend on the temperature increase induced by the laser energy delivered to the irradiated area and the exposure time. In addition the degree of uniformity of the tissue concerned and the extent to which it is perfused with blood also considerably affect the temperature reached and its consequences. Finally, one of the most important elements to take into account is whether the effects on the tissue are reversible or not – irreversible damage corresponds to effective necrosis.

A temperature-dependent scale to describe the effect of heat on living tissue can be drawn up *(tables I and II)*. From a clinical point of view, tissue damage is induced *via* three distinct mechanisms, namely hyperthermia (at temperatures of between 41 and 44°C), coagulation (between 50 and 90°C) and vaporisation (at over 100°C).

■ The thermal effect of 810 nm diode lasers

One of the main preoccupations in laser therapy is to minimise the damage mediated by the laser shot and to restrict it as far as possible to the irradiated area, *i.e.* the target zone. This is a particularly important consideration in neurosurgery given the functional importance and fragility of nearby cerebral and medullary tissues. For this reason, it seemed essential to perform complementary experiments on animals in order to compare the effects of the different laser models that we have been (over the past 15 years) and are still using for neurosurgical applications in humans. The aim of these experiments was to provide neurosurgeons who use high-power lasers (whether it be regularly or occasionally) with accurate information on the effects induced by the following common types of neurosurgical laser: CO_2, 1.06 μm Nd-YAG, 1.32 μm Nd-YAG and 810 nm diode. These studies were conducted using the brains of rats and rabbits and samples of human tissue taken during operations.

	Table I
41 to 44° C	**Hyperthermia**
50 to 90° C	**Coagulation**
> 100° C	**Vaporisation, sectioning**

Table II
The effects of temperature on living tissue

Temperature (° C)	Effect on tissue
45	**Vasodilatation** **Endothelial lesions** Cell death
50	All enzyme activity blocked
57	Conversion of proteins
60	**Denaturation of proteins** Loss of membrane structure
70	**Denaturation of collagen** Permeabilisation of membranes
80	Contraction of collagen **Coagulation necrosis**
100	Vaporisation of water Generation of steam Complete dehydration
> 100	**Vaporisation** Cell fragmentation Carbonisation
200 to 300	Appearance of smoke
500 to 600	Incandescence

These studies conducted using the laser in a "free-beam" or "non-contact" mode showed that the effects of 810 nm diode lasers were comparable to those of 1.06 µm Nd-YAG lasers in terms of thermal damage. However, the action of diode lasers is actually more localised because of higher levels of thermal absorption and lower tissue penetration so in the final analysis it acts more like the 1.32 µm Nd-YAG laser. Therefore, **diode lasers induce haemostasis in a similar way to 1.06 µm Nd-YAG lasers but, in terms of sectioning and vaporisation, their action is more like that of 1.32 µm Nd-YAG lasers.**

The optical penetration of a laser beam incident on living tissue depends on the percentage of the radiation which is reflected compared with the proportion which is absorbed in the specific tissue under consideration. **Absorption and diffusion are the means whereby the electromagnetic energy of laser light is converted into heat, a conversion process which is extremely wavelength-dependent.** The infrared radiation emitted by an 810 nm laser is only absorbed very weakly by water, protein and nucleic acids but, in contrast, it is strongly absorbed by pigment molecules such as melanin, haemoglobin, myoglobin and bilirubin.

■ In practice, in nervous tissue which contains high proportions of water and lipids, diffusion of the ray is of the order of 20 to 30% in the white matter and of 30 to 40% in the grey matter; absorption is virtually zero in the former and of the order of about 10% in the latter. In tumour tissue, absorption is more efficient and it increases with the extent of vascularization of the tumour, e.g. highly vascular masses like meningiomas and high grade gliomas absorb 810 nm radiation efficiently and, in theory, coagulation of such tumours can be achieved relatively easily using a diode laser. On the other hand, in relatively avascular and unpigmented tissue like the spinal cord and oedematous cerebral parenchyma, 810 nm diode lasers are poorly effective for haemostasis.

Lasers and safety

Nothing in this chapter is specific to diode lasers but anyone using any type of laser in medicine or surgery should be familiar with the main hazards associated with their use in the operating theatre and all the various safety precautions which should be taken.

■ Hazards and safety precautions

The rate of occurrence of accidents or other types of incidents during surgical procedures involving lasers being performed in operating theatres is of the order of three for every 1,000 interventions. The two organs most commonly at risk in such accidents are the eyes and the skin.

■ The risk to the eyes

The radiation emitted by diode lasers is in the infrared range, like that of CO_2 and Nd-YAG lasers. Whether the wavelength of the beam is 810 nm (the Diomed laser) or 1,000 nm, the components of the eye which are most at risk are the retina, the lens and the cornea with the most common complications being *cataract* and *burning of the retina*. In the worst-case scenario, a single exposure of the fovea centralis to the beam could lead to total blindness in the exposed eye *(table III)*. In reality, the risk of this happening is extremely small because the beam would either have to be deliberately directed or reflected off an instrument straight into somebody's eye. Nevertheless, this risk, albeit small, means that everybody present in the operating theatre must, at all times, wear *safety glasses* specially designed to block the relevant wavelength. If an operating microscope is being used, it should be fitted with a *special filter* between the objective lens and the body of the instrument. This is all the more important because such magnifying instruments focus the beam thereby also magnifying the danger to the eyes. Appropriate

	Table III Potential laser-mediated damage to the eyes						
Wavelength (nm)	UV(C) 200-280	UV(B) 280-315	UV(A) 315-400	Visible 400-780	IR(A) 780-1,400	IR(B) 1,400-3,000	IR(C) 3,000-10,000
Structure affected	Cornea	Cornea	Cornea Lens Retina		Cornea Lens Retina	Cornea Lens	Cornea
Pathology	Keratitis	Keratitis	Conjunctivitis Cataract		Cataract Burning of the retina	Cataract Burning of the cornea	Burning of the cornea

filters are permanently mounted on our operating microscopes. Of course, anyone actually working with the microscope, be it the surgeon or his or her assistant, does not need to wear safety glasses because they are already being protected by the filter in the microscope. In order to cut down the risk of the beam getting reflected off instruments, it is preferable if not essential to try to use *non-shiny instruments* whenever possible. When a shaped fibre is being used, the risk to the eyes is zero because the laser beam is only concentrated and focused at the very tip of the fibre optic.

■ The risk to the skin

After the eye, the organ which is the next most likely to be damaged by laser radiation is the skin. As is obvious, the seriousness of this danger does not compare with that of the danger to the eyes and, in addition, in contrast to the retina, damaged skin heals quite rapidly so the consequences of exposure would also usually be less serious. If the beam strikes a gloved hand at an angle, the latex will heat up and in some cases a blister might be raised on the underlying skin. If it strikes perpendicularly, a hole might be burnt in the glove and the underlying skin will be burnt, the deepness of the burn depending on a variety of factors.

The extent of damage to the skin will depend on the wavelength of the beam and on its absorption by the pigments and water in the cutaneous tissue. Concerning the 810 nm wavelength, there is absorption by both melanin and haemoglobin. The level of absorption is such that exposure to the continuous laser beam would cause a subcutaneous burn.

■ Precautions

In practice, all these problems are rare and can be avoided by implementing simple precautionary measures and safety rules.

A warning notice should be displayed on the door to the operating theatre:

> Danger – Laser in operation
> SAFETY GLASSES **MUST** BE WORN

Ideally, the access point to any room in which a laser is in operation should be fitted with a luminous sign. Whenever a laser is actually in operation, the number of people present in the theatre should be kept to a minimum and everyone inside MUST be wearing *protective safety glasses* which are appropriate for the wavelength and power rating of the laser in use. These glasses must be within EN 207 and 208 specifications. Whenever the laser is not in use, the key to its control panel should be kept in a safe place so that no unauthorised personnel can touch it.

The safety of lasers is also dependent on how well they are maintained. Maintenance operations should only be performed by specially trained technicians. In a similar vein, the training of all operating theatre personnel is very important, whether it be the surgeons themselves or ancillary staff.

■ National and international regulations

Each different country has its own specific approach to regulating and accrediting lasers for medical use. Differences were particularly marked between different European countries until European Union (EU) Directives were issued stipulating a common set of norms governing the labelling and certification of equipment to be applied across the board in all member states. It should be noted, however, that rapid progress in laser techniques and increasing integration of computers into procedures has led to ever more complicated protocols in recent years.

The International Electric Commission (IEC) compiled norm 601-1 in 1977 concerning "Electromedical Devices. General Safety Rules" which is applicable to a wide variety of different types of device including lasers. This norm, together with the later IEC 820 ("Electrical Safety of Devices and Laser Equipment") and IEC 825

("Safety of Laser Radiation, Classification of Equipment, Prescription and User's Guide), stipulate norms for safety, the construction of machines, precautions against electric shocks, the risks associated with undesirable irradiation, the risk of explosion, leakage currents, etc. This set of norms is not applicable in either Canada or the USA.

The relationship between accreditation and forensic liability is clear in terms of the Penal Code, civil law and government regulations. The certificate of accreditation affords the director of any hospital buying a piece of equipment a guarantee that the machine has been well built and is of a certain standard of quality. It gives him the confirmation that the choice of the specific device was motivated and justified in terms of the regulations in force. Subsequently, it is the facility which is responsible for the maintenance and proper working of the laser device in the same way as it is responsible for the operating theatre and all its accessories which are subject to very strict regulations. Accreditation of all the devices used according to European norms should also be considered as a means of protecting the manufacturer. Insofar as the surgeon is concerned, analysis of the relevant case law shows that the best way to guard against potential malpractice suits related to the medical use of lasers is to undergo all the special training necessary in the use of this type of instrument. This is why we attach so much importance to training in all its forms and especially if it results in some kind of concrete qualification.

■ Training and education

Without going into details about what exactly a laser training course includes or should include, we would like to outline a few general principles.

Until very recently, the only real opportunity for training which was available was to work side by side with an experienced operator, which was true for both surgeons and ancillary operating theatre personnel. However, more recently, specific courses and seminars have begun to appear, first in the United States and later in Europe. Such courses help round off the knowledge acquired by working together with experienced operators and at conferences.

To us, it seems very important that such formal, recognised courses should exist in order to respond to the need which is ever more increasingly felt for validated training courses and forensic liability on the part of the users of special surgical equipment.

The teaching of how to use laser technology in medicine and surgery should fulfil certain general principles including: a) rational educational methods, b) the use of simulations, c) some kind of evaluation procedure, of both student and teacher, d) the creation and development of centres of experimentation and training, e) the development of multimedia-based materials designed for training.

Technical data

■ Semiconductor diode lasers

Here we will describe the **Diomed 30** model which comprises a series of **Aluminium / Gallium Arsenide (Ga Al As) diodes** and which emits at **a wavelength of 810 ± 25 nm** in the **infrared range** of the electromagnetic spectrum. This was the first commercially available semiconductor laser of high enough power for surgical applications. For a preliminary period of one year we tried out and tested this machine in the context of its accreditation, mainly for France and Europe. We have been routinely using it since 1993 for certain neurosurgical procedures which we will describe in detail in the next chapter.

This **portable machine** has dimensions of 40 x 38.15 cm and weighs 11 kg. It does not need any kind of cooling system and putting it into operation is extremely simple – it simply has to be connected to the main power supply (110/220 V) and the starter key activated. Its compact size means that it is easy to transport from one operating theatre to another or even, if necessary, from one hospital to another in its custom-made metal box.

It consists of a **housing which contains a generator**, *i.e.* an array of diodes. On the front of the machine is a **control panel** with three adjustable dials **for regulating the main parameters**, *i.e.* power output, exposure time and the length of time between pulses. In addition, there are three digital buttons which give simple, fast access to the main menu from which the choice of continuous or pulsed operation can be made, the machine can be put on stand-by and other functions like calibration, statistical data and calibration checking can be accessed. The controls are very user-friendly so all members of the operating theatre team learn to use them very quickly, both in terms of installation and operation *(figure 12)*.

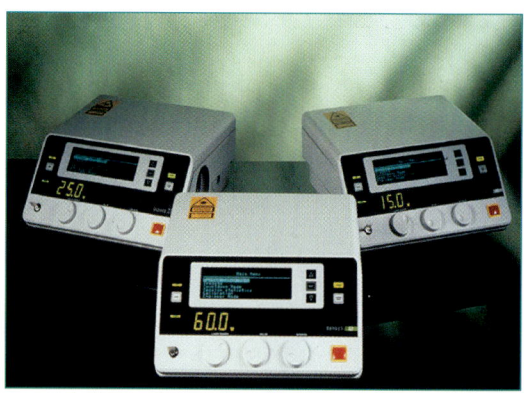

Figure 12. *The Diomed semiconductor diode laser.*

The model of the machine we have used has a maximum **power output** rating of 30 W to the fibre port. The laser beam can be either a continuous or pulsed beam (t = 100 msec; F = 10 Hz) with a frequency ranging from 0.1 second to 1 second. There are also two other laser options, the Diomed 15 which emits a maximum of 15 W cw and the Diomed 60 which emits up to 60 W. These different models can all be used with either **quartz fibre optic** (with diameters of 400, 600 and 1,000 µm) **in non-contact mode** or with **shaped fibres for use in contact mode** *(figure 13)*. The latter are available with either a 300 µm conical tip or with a spherical tip of either 800 or 1,000 µm. The diameter of the actual fibre (for both conical and spherical tips) can be of either 600 or 1,000 µm. All fibres are for single use only and are 3 metres in length. Non-contact fibres can be fitted onto a hand piece which is slim and autoclavable. The hand piece has a diameter of 9 millimetres and is either 61 or 113 millimetres in length. There are two different types of adapter. One type is soft, flexible and telescopic (going from 2.5 to 11 cm) which means that its shape and length can be easily changed during a procedure as needs dictate; this is the type of adapter which we prefer to use because it is often better suited to neurosurgical applications. The other type of adapter is rigid and is of fixed length (either, 2.5, 5, 11 or 35 cm). For endoscopy, it is clearly better to use non-contact fibres which can be inserted into the endoscope's working channel. All these various types of fibre can be connected to the control panel *via* a standard SMA-905 connector.

Among the many advantages of diode lasers, we would emphasise the fact that they require very little maintenance. The lifetime of the diodes is of the order of 10 to 20,000 hours which means that any machine can be used for something like 60,000 interventions given that, in the course of a neurosurgical procedure, a laser is rarely operated for more than 10 to 20 minutes in real time.

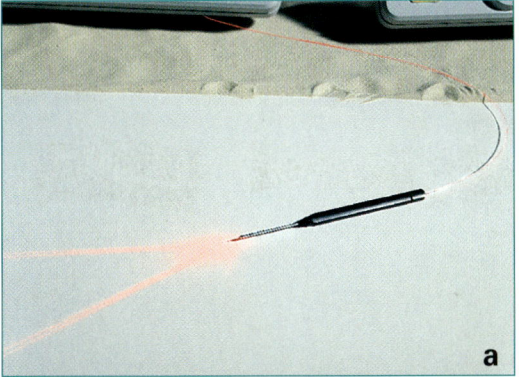
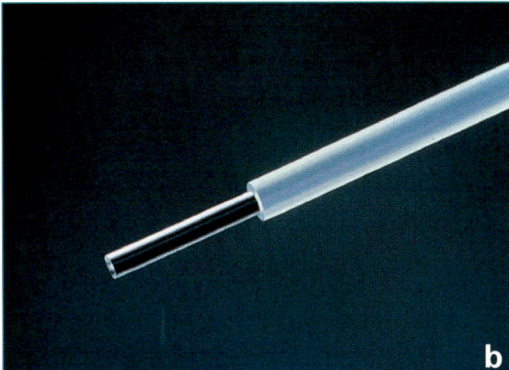
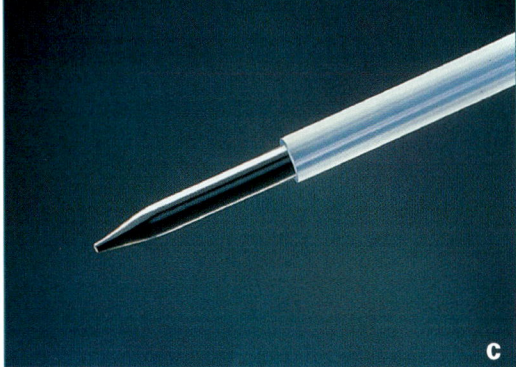

■ **Figure 13**. *Accessories for a diode laser:*
a) hand piece;
b) non-contact bare end fibre (diameter = 400 μm);
c) shaped fibre for contact mode (diameter = 600 μm).

■ Techniques in neurosurgery: general principles

As described above, the radiation emitted by diode lasers is efficiently absorbed by both pigmented and vascularized tissue. This is why it is such a useful instrument for operating on most of the tumours involved in neurosurgery and why it is so effective for haemostasis in the course of common procedures which involve intracranial or intraspinal interventions, whether it is being used in non-contact mode or in contact mode with a shaped fibre. Similarly, tissues can be readily vaporised with a non-contact fibre as long as sufficiently high power outputs are used (10 to 25 W, preferably in pulsed operation). Thus, as has already been mentioned, the surgical properties of 810 nm diode lasers are highly comparable to those of 1.32 μm Nd-YAG lasers.

■ From the outset, one important point is worth underlining: **how to obtain a given effect on tissue can be ascertained very quickly by adjusting the different laser emission parameters, whatever the machine's specific wavelength. This means that it is always possible to obtain the desired action, be it coagulation, sectioning or vaporisation**, by either focusing the beam or putting it out of focus, by increasing or decreasing output power, or by switching between continuous and pulsed operation.

■ In conjunction with Cavitron UltraSound Aspiration (CUSA)

In the next chapter, it will be seen how the use of lasers is tightly associated with CUSA in a variety of neurosurgical procedures, in particular interventions in the posterior cranial fossa and the spinal cord. Together with lasers, ultrasound aspirators are members of the group of "non-touch technique" devices which can be used to avoid or reduce causing mechanical injury to functionally important central nervous system structures.

■ Non-contact mode

■ Volatilisation: vaporisation and sectioning

The process of vaporisation corresponds to the sudden loss of substance which occurs when the temperature of the target area is elevated to over 100° C for a short period of time (of between a few microseconds to a few tenths of a second). The tissue struck by the laser radiation is converted into steam. Depending on the temperature reached, the vaporisation process involves different stages and can progress through charring and combustion, and ultimately to sublimation.

If the area of the target tissue is sufficiently large (of the order of millimetres), sudden elevation of the temperature to high levels will result in its vaporisation. In practice, for this, the laser power output has to be of the order of 10 to 25 W in either cw or pulsed mode – pulsed mode is more efficient because the peak output values are higher and it is the preferable mode of emission for firm tumours like meningiomas.

If the target area is smaller (less than one millimetre), the result will be the sectioning of the tissue. This can be used to fragment large tumours but, nevertheless, it has become clear that using a laser alone is not the best way to fragment any large tumour, whether it be a meningioma, a schwannoma or any other kind, because it takes too long. Rather, preliminary fragmentation should be undertaken using conventional instruments or the CUSA and then the laser can be used to vaporise the deeper fragments. The diode laser really comes into its own when residual tumoral fragments need to be removed and when relatively small tumours are located close to functionally important areas (*e.g.* in the posterior cranial fossa or the spinal cord).

During vaporisation, significant amounts of steam are generated. Therefore, as mentioned in chapter 5, it is essential to provide an adequately powerful aspiration system with a probe which can be positioned very close to the impact point of the laser beam. This system should also be fitted with an appropriate filter. Finally, suction apparatus based on plastic materials which might melt or burst into flames must be excluded – only apparatus made of glass or non-shiny metal should be used.

Haemostasis

As mentioned above, coagulation is achieved by maintaining a temperature of near 80° C for a period of about one second. This exposure induces tissue retraction as a consequence of the local denaturation of proteins.

The high temperature associated with photocoagulation actually induces denaturation of plasma proteins, retraction of the collagen in vessel walls and damage to endothelial tissue and erythrocytes. All this damage leads to the sealing off of the lumen of any vessels struck by the laser beam, which effect results from a combination of different factors: a) the slowing down of blood flow caused by an increase in viscosity, b) a shrinking of the blood vessel, and c) the activation and aggregation of platelets. Actual haemostasis is consequent on the formation of an area of coagulation necrosis and retraction of the vessel walls. Obviously, such coagulation necrosis should not be associated with any vaporisation of the target tissue or of any local blood vessels, which would only tend to exacerbate the bleeding which is what the process is supposed to be preventing in the first place. Superficial coagulation (to a depth of about one millimetre) is adequate for capillary haemostasis but, to coagulate an arteriole of 2 mm in diameter, the laser beam and/or thermal diffusion will have to penetrate to a depth of at least three millimetres.

From a practical point of view, haemostasis is achieved with the diode laser operating continuously, with a beam that can either be highly focused "less than 10 mm from the target" or relatively out of focus (1-2 cm from the target), and at a power output of between 3 and 10 W. The softer the target tissue and the smaller the vessels concerned, the lower the power output necessary. As will be seen later, haemostasis of the insertion point of a meningioma can be readily achieved with a relatively low-power beam (5 to 8 W) unless the lumens of the meningeal vessels concerned are of one millimetre or more in diameter. If such is the case, it will be necessary either to increase the power output of the laser or, as is often required to avoid wasting time and ensure effective haemostasis, resort to bipolar or perhaps unipolar electrocoagulation. When a meningioma is inserted into bone tissue, it may be necessary to increase the power output to char the bone itself.

■ Contact mode

With contact fibres, the issues are somewhat different. In this case, the laser radiation is concentrated at the end of the shaped tip which gives the capacity for sectioning without any diffusion of heat. As will be explained later, this also means efficient haemostasis of the sectioned surface. On the other hand, emission parameters cannot be varied to anything like the same extent because, as was mentioned above, high power output and the consequent elevated temperatures might cause melting of the shaped tip – in our experience, it is better to avoid power output levels of over 10 W (5 to 8 W is a safe range) and always operate in continuous mode *(table IV)*.

To avoid diffusion of laser energy from the end of the fibre and to increase power density, it is recommended to carbonise the fibre tip either by placing it in contact with blood or a wooden spatula at a laser energy of 10 W.

Table IV
Power output levels used for function of desired tissue effects

	Haemostasis	Sectioning	Vaporisation
Contact (shaped fibres)	cw: 3-8 W	cw: 5-10 W	N/A
Non-contact	cw: 3-10 W	cw/p: 10-20 W	p: 15-25 W

cw: continuous mode; p: pulsed mode.

■ Minimally invasive neurosurgery (MIN)

Minimally invasive neurosurgery has been developing at a rapid pace in recent years as the understanding and the methods of stereotactic surgery have improved, notably due to progress in the fields of computer-assisted techniques and high resolution, digitised medical imaging. This trend can only continue to accelerate with the establishment of more interventional navigation units in neurosurgery operating theatres. It is easy to imagine that, in 5 to 10 years from now, *i.e.* by 2005 to 2010, most neurosurgery departments will be in possession of such equipment, with or without associated robotic systems. Any kind of device or machine which makes minimally invasive procedures easier obviously has a place during such procedures, including fibre optic-compatible lasers in general and diode lasers in particular. The recognised advantages of minimally invasive stereotactic techniques are the need for very small cranial openings, a reduction in iatrogenic injuries to encephalic and intraspinal structures, reductions in morbidity and mortality, and, as a result, the cutting of health care costs. Intracranial endoscopy also provides parallel benefits.

■ Stereotactic surgery

Ever since the beginning of the 1980's, Patrick Kelly has pioneered combining lasers with stereotactic methods and, more recently, he has been important in the development of ways of associating interventional navigation and robotics with the integration of CT and MRI data and peroperative data management systems. Great advances have been made in two main areas, namely: 1) stereotactically guided surgery and 2) interventional navigation systems, whether robotic or not.

■ Stereotactically guided surgery

Such techniques allow intracranial surgery *via* very small openings with stereotactic guiding systems coupled with CT scanning or MRI and sometimes arteriography. These methods depend on a stereotactic frame fixed to the patient's skull. This apparatus functions as both an external geometrical reference for calculating the spatial co-ordinates of any given point inside the skull and also for holding and guiding the surgical instruments being used. The approach routes to be used during the operation are simulated using computer-assisted image-processing which allows the size of holes made in the skull to be reduced to the minimum necessary for any planned operation. These holes are usually round craniotomies of between just 20 and 40 mm, which expose only a tiny fraction of the brain's surface.

By virtue of their great manoeuvrability and small bulk, lasers are ideal instruments for use in the very confined spaces involved in these minimally invasive procedures. Diode lasers used in contact mode can be used to resect superficial, cortical and sub-cortical lesions (metastases or small meningiomas) with little concomitant injury to surrounding tissues and with clean, haemostatic dissection of the tumour away from the neighbouring, healthy cerebral tissue.

■ Interventional navigation

Interventional navigation represents an advance in the techniques of stereotactically guided surgery in the sense that real-time imaging is used to monitor the progress of the operation. The stereotactic frame is no longer necessary to acquire the CT and MRI images. Surgical navigation is taken care of by instruments fitted with infrared LEDs, the position of which can be monitored in real time by special detectors. The end of the instrument is shown on the corresponding CT or MRI images thus telling the surgeon exactly where the instrument is located in relation to the various cerebral structures and the lesion to be excised. The "navigating" instrument can be a simple pointer, dissecting forceps, an endoscope or the hand piece of a fibre optic laser. Interventional navigation seems to be one of the most effective minimally invasive techniques currently in use because, on the one hand, the pointer can be used to target the best route for the surgical instruments and, on the other hand, because of the reduced size of the craniotomies necessary to perform the operations. The use of diode laser fibres in conjunction with these techniques (when possible and worthwhile) obviously consolidates the non-invasiveness of such procedures and helps further reduce concomitant injury to healthy tissue.

Neuroendoscopy

We will deal in detail with the use of diode lasers in endoscopy in the next chapter.

It is obvious that the only type of fibre which can be used is a bare end non-contact one with the appropriate diameter for the endoscope's working channel. We usually use **600 μm fibres with an output power of between 4 and 6 W cw**. The virtue of radiation at 805 nm is that it is not absorbed by water molecules and therefore the cerebrospinal fluid (CSF) which fills ventricular cavities is transparent to it. As a result, it is possible to coagulate or section the capsule of a tumour or a cyst by placing the fibre either in contact with it or very close (within 1 to 2 mm).

The two main indications are: 1) colloid cysts in the third ventricle and 2) performing ventriculocisternostomies. We have also used the same equipment to help excise and biopsy intraventricular tumours like meningiomas and gliomas.

For colloid cysts, laser fibres can be used to bypass certain difficult peroperative manipulations, in particular to open the walls of very solid cysts. In this case, the target is coagulated at 4 or 5 W cw and then incised with a slightly higher power output but operating in pulsed mode with the tip of the fibre in direct contact. Objectively speaking, the wavelength of 810 nm is not the only one suitable for this type of procedure and, in fact, both types of Nd-YAG laser (1.06 and 1.32 µm) which we have been using for over 10 years now have proven extremely effective in the removal of such cysts.

In all these examples in which laser radiation is being used in ventricular cavities (and especially when operating near the anterior columns of the fornix of cerebrum), it is vital to avoid misdirecting the beam because of the risk of inducing thermal damage and causing postoperative complications with memory function. This is why all irradiation should be carried out in contact mode or at least very close to the target, be it a cyst, a tumour or the basal third ventricle in the case of ventriculocisternostomies.

Neurosurgical applications for diode lasers

■ Intracranial tumour

■ The types of intracranial tumour which are most suitable for laser-assisted ablation are the benign forms, especially the various meningiomas (wherever they are localised). In addition, lasers, and in particular diode lasers, can be useful for gaining access to lesions involving the brain stem and for removing acoustic neuromas. As will be explained later, diode lasers can be easily and successfully used in conjunction with ultrasound cavitation (CUSA). Of course, these tumours do not represent the only ones which can be treated with diode lasers but, in our opinion, they are the most obviously amenable.

■ Meningiomas

Supratentorial convexity tumours

- **If the meningioma is large** (over 4 cm in diameter), it should not be removed in one piece but should rather be first dissected into smaller fragments. There are various different ways of going about this:

1. If a Nd-YAG 1.06 µm laser is available, the tumour should first be partly dehydrated by heating which both shrinks the tumour mass and facilitates access to the plane of dissection between meningioma and the cerebral cortex. Then the tumour can be dissected using conventional instruments like scissors together with a **diode laser in contact mode**. In these examples, we recommend using a **1,000 µm shaped fibre** with a relatively high power setting to guarantee effective cutting (10 to 20 W in continuous mode [cw]). Smaller fibres are more fragile and are not designed to be used at these high powers.

2. If no YAG laser is available, the first step is to coagulate the capsule using either the diode laser in non-contact mode (with a fibre of 400 to 600 µm and a power setting of 8 to 10 W in cw) or bipolar electrocoagulation. An incision should be made in the capsule using a 1,000 µm sculpted fibre at a power of 10 to 20 W (cw). Dissection can then be performed as described above.

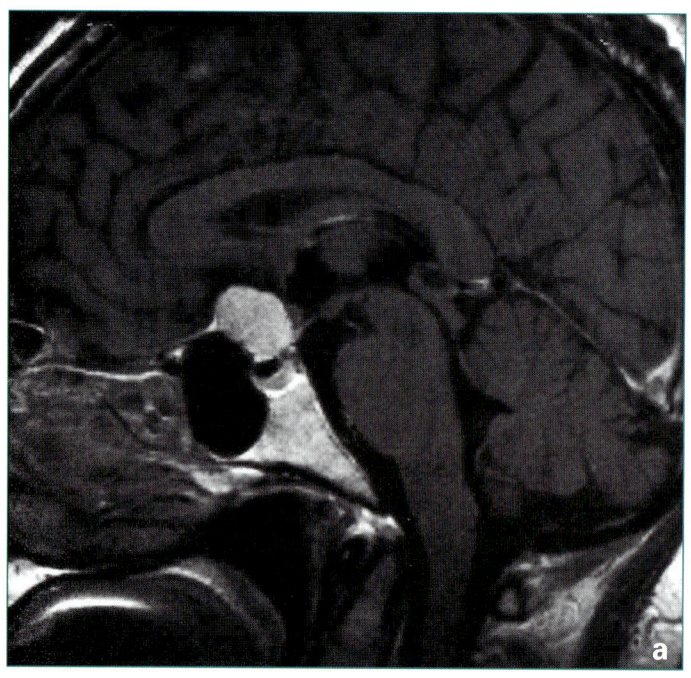

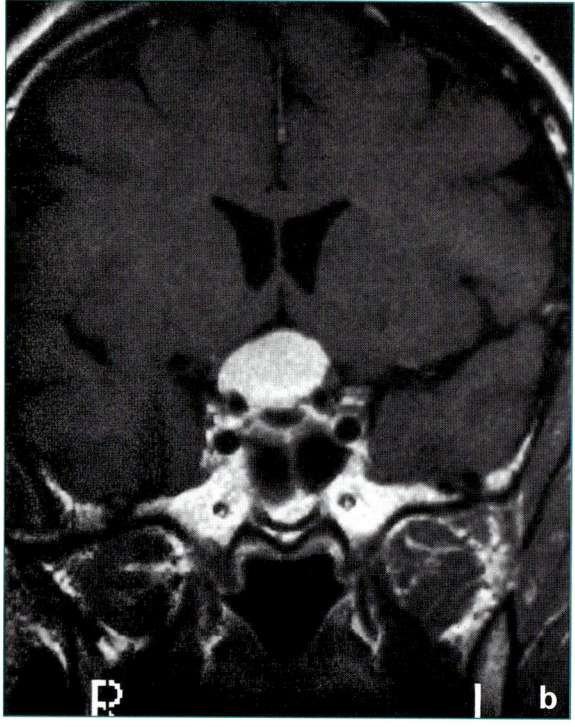

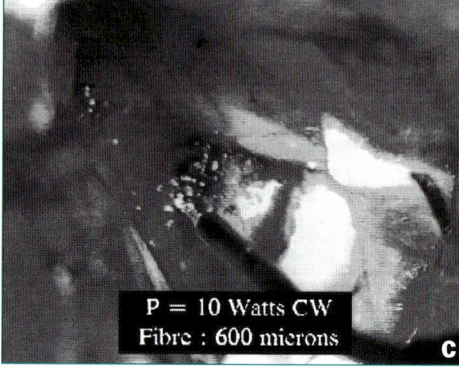

■ **Figure 14.** A meningioma of the jugum in a 49 year-old woman which manifested as a bilateral loss of visual acuity.
a, b) Preoperative MRI, T1 after injection of gadolinium.
c, Peroperative view. The diode laser is being operated in non-contact mode with a 600 μm fibre and at a power output of 10 W in pulsed mode to perforate the capsule and section the insertion base.

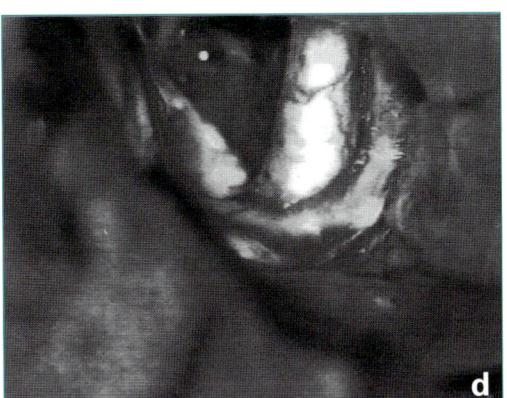
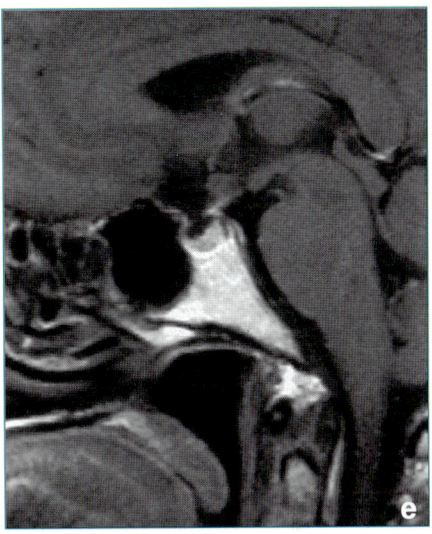
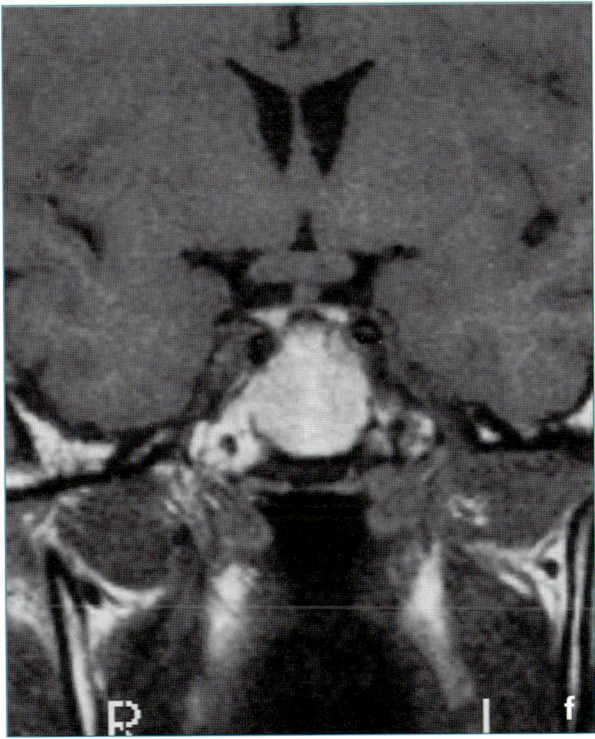

d) Peroperative view. By the end of the operation, the tumour has been completely excised. Both optic nerves (NO) have been relieved and released throughout their length, as has been the right internal carotid artery (outside of the right optic nerve) in its extra-cavernous portion. The anterior cerebral artery can also be seen crossing the upper side of the right optic nerve.
e, f) Postoperative MRI confirming that removal of the tumour was complete: both the optic nerves and the pituitary stalk are completely free.

3) If a cavitron ultrasound aspirator (CUSA) is available (as is the case in most operating theatres used for neurosurgery these days), dissection of the tumour will be much easier if the tumour is not too firm. In this case, a diode laser can be used to coagulate and section tumour capillaries as they are exposed. In order to coagulate these capillaries, the surgeon can choose to operate in either contact mode (a 400 to 600 µm bare end fibre with a power of 8-12 W cw) or non-contact mode with the same parameters as above.

Never persist with laser diode-assisted haemostasis (or coagulation with any other kind of laser) if it is proving difficult – bipolar coagulation is often more effective. **Using a laser should NEVER result in the prolongation of any procedure**.

- **If the tumour is small**, it can often be dissected out and cleanly enucleated in which case using a diode laser is not advantageous. However, if the tumour is located in a dangerous area, an operating microscope can be used to guide the laser beam with pinpoint accuracy and the surrounding, healthy tissue can be protected with cottonoid. This is most relevant to the anatomical locations described below, namely the posterior cranial fossa and the base of the skull.

Meningiomas involving the anterior base of the skull

One of the first surgeons to highlight the value of lasers in the ablation of meningiomas located at the base of the skull was A.D. Bartal in Tel Aviv in 1982.

Among the best targets for diode laser-assisted surgery at the base of the skull are suprasellar meningiomas *(figure 14)* and meningiomas of the sphenoid ridge. Both these types of tumour are closely associated with the carotid artery and its branches and optic nerve structures (the optic nerve itself and the optic chiasm), as is also true for meningiomas of the olfactory groove *(figure 15)*. In all of these cases, it is important to first reduce the volume of the tumour, either using conventional methods, ultrasound cavitation or a diode laser in contact mode (with a 600 or 1,000 µm shaped fibre and a power setting of 10 W cw).

Subsequently, using an optical magnification system, any fragments of the tumour located near or on the optic nerve or the internal carotid artery and its branches have to be removed. This can be achieved using either contact or non-contact mode but we prefer the former.

- **For contact mode**, we recommend a 600 µm conical shaped fibre with low power – of the order of only 5 to 8 W because of the proximity of the optic nerve and important blood vessels like the internal carotid artery, and the origins of the middle and/or anterior cerebral arteries.

- **In non-contact mode**, pulses should be of short duration, of the order of one second. The beam should be as focused as possible, *i.e.* the laser fibre held at less than 10 mm from the target, and pulses can be repeated as often as is necessary as long as very low power is used (less than 5 W) in order to protect underlying anatomical structures. The value of using repeated, short pulses lies in the fact that any heat generated dissipates during the relaxation time between each pulse thereby reducing the risk of inducing thermal damage to the underlying tissue.

We have already mentioned the reasons for using the laser to char the insertion point of a meningioma, whether it is purely meningeal in nature or whether it is also involving bone tissue. For this, a 400 or 600 µm bare end non-contact fibre should be used with adequate power output (at least 10 to 15 W). Given the amount of smoke which is given off during such an exercise, adequate aspiration must be provided in order to keep the operator's field of vision clear.

If the meningioma has grown into the cavernous sinus, we recommend that the infiltration be sterilised by scanning with a 400 or 600 µm fibre at a power output of 10 to 12 W cw. It is best to put the beam slightly out of focus in order to cut down the risk of damaging healthy tissue.

Meningiomas of the sphenoid ridge

The advantages of diode lasers in this case are the same as those mentioned above in the context of meningiomas located at the anterior base of the skull. However, the fact that these tumours often infiltrate bone tissue should be borne in mind. Charring infiltrated bone tissue can be worthwhile in that recurrence may be delayed as suggested by certain studies into the recurrence of laser-treated meningiomas (O.J. Beck, 1980). Such charring can be achieved using a non-contact 1,000 µm fibre at a relatively high power output (15 to 20 W in pulsed mode).

Meningiomas of the posterior cranial fossa, the petro-clival region and the foramen magnum

Posterior cranial fossa surgery has been veritably transformed by the use of a combination of lasers and the CUSA. This is particularly true for meningiomas and bulky schwannomas. Significant reductions in

■ Diode lasers in neurosurgery

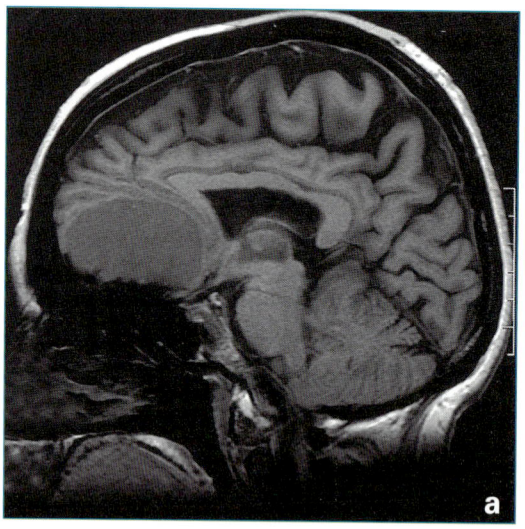
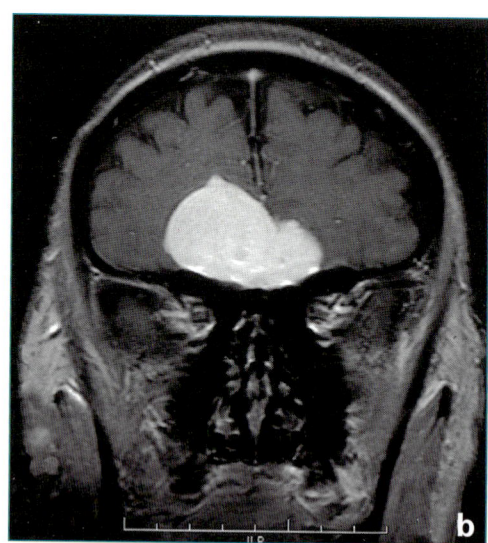
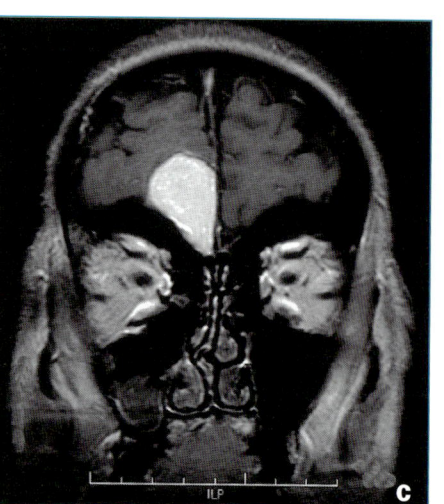
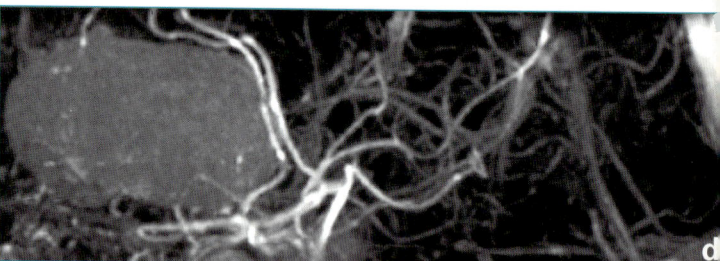
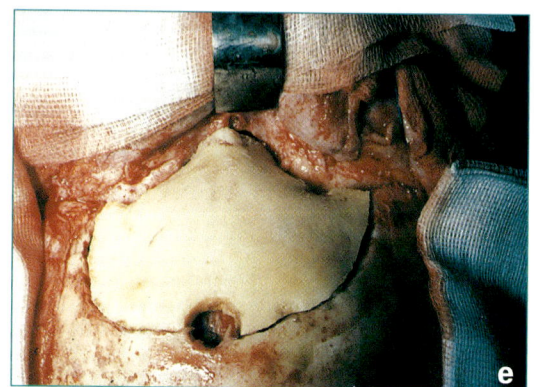

■ **Figure 15.** *An olfactory meningioma in a 45 year-old woman which manifested as preferential anosmia.*
a, b, c) Preoperative MRI and d) AngioMRI.
e, f, g) Surgical sub-fronto-orbito-nasal approach.
h, i, j) Dissection and progressive release of optic nerves using a conical shaped fibre (600 μm) in contact mode with a laser output power of 8 W cw.
k, l) Postoperative follow-up CT scan (performed immediately after the intervention) confirming that the tumour has been completely excised. The patient was discharged eight days after the operation.

Neurosurgical applications

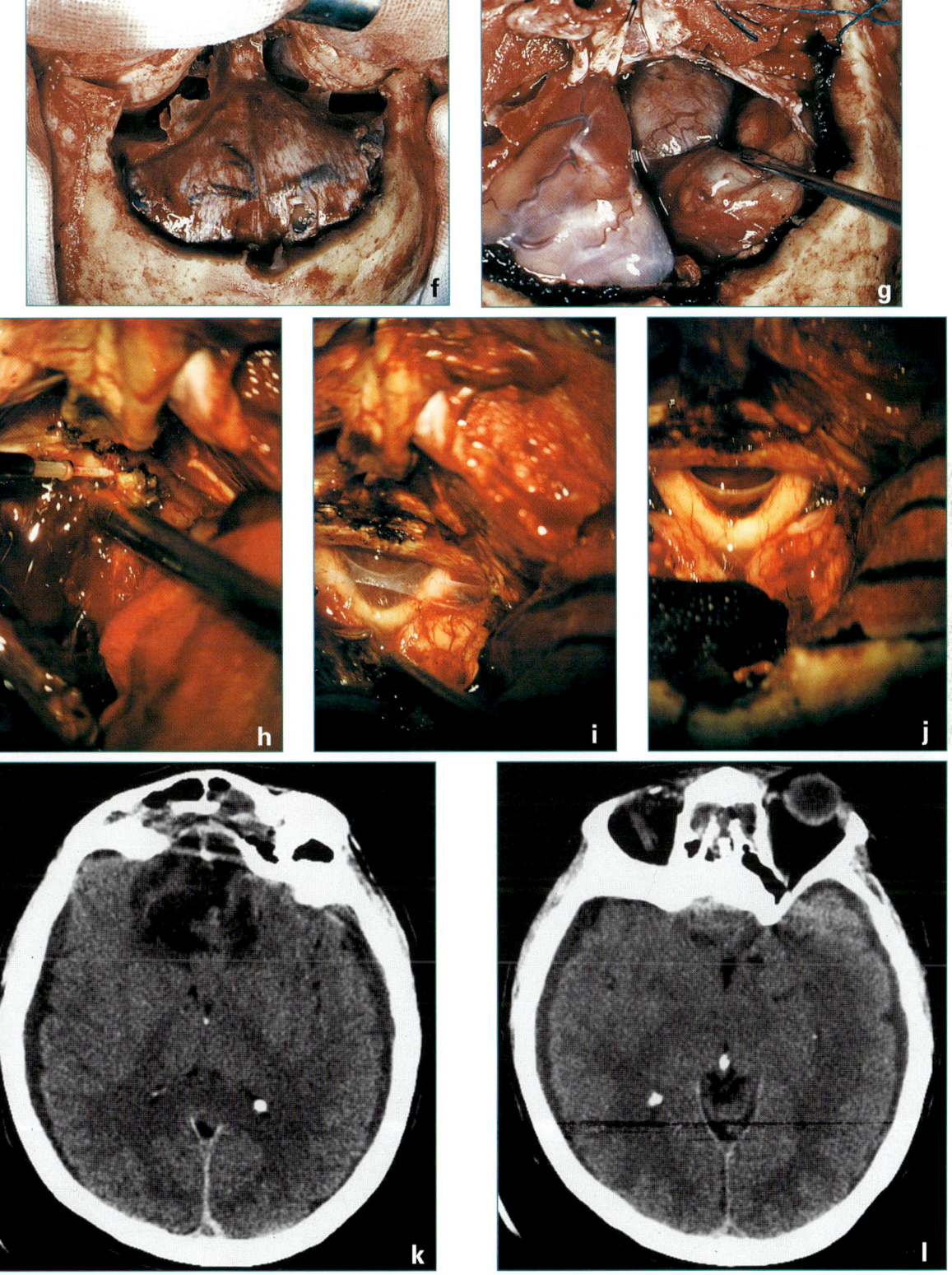

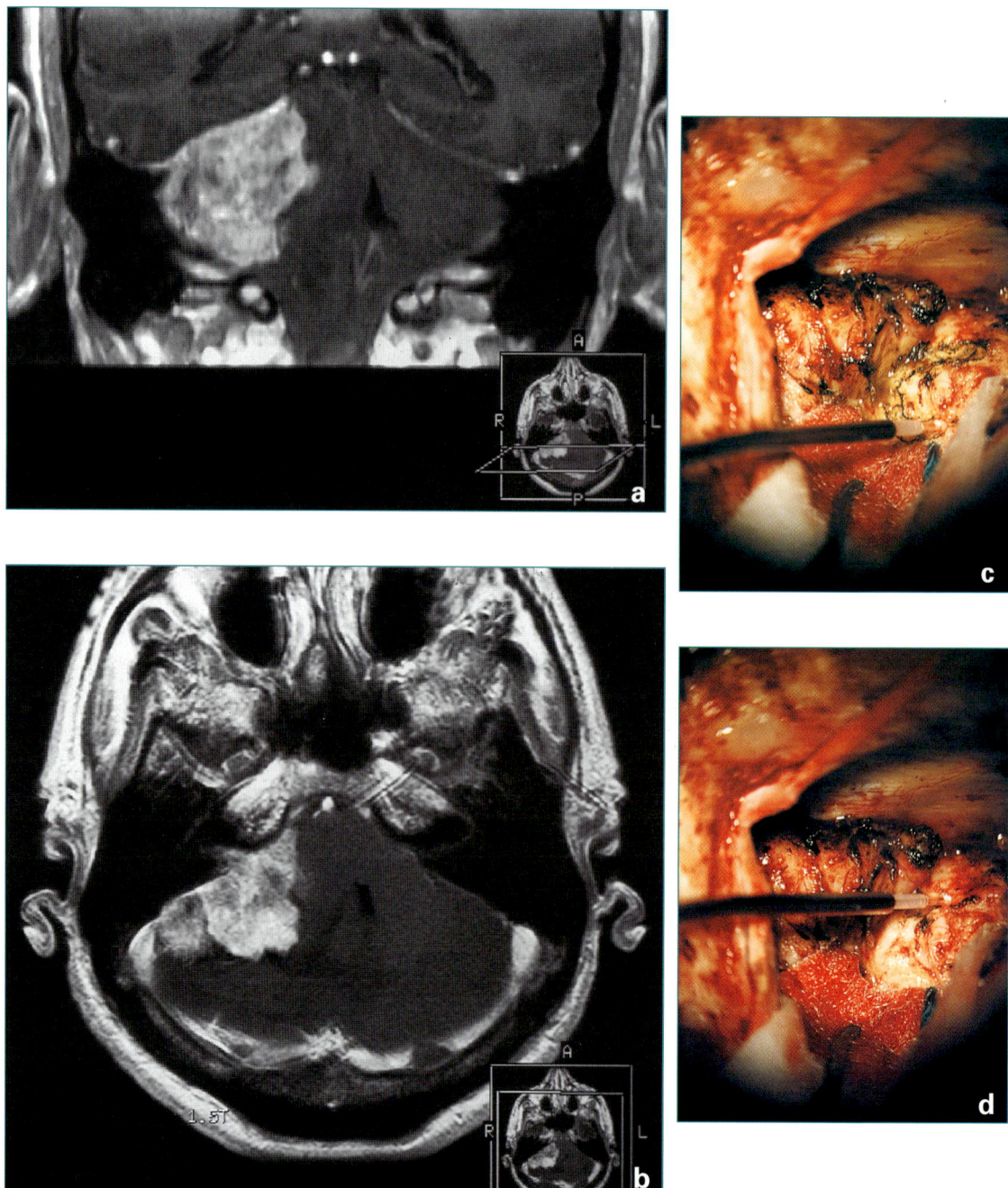

Figure 16. Meningioma of the posterior cranial fossa in a 60 year-old man. Inserted into the lower side of the tentorium cerebelli and the posterior intracranial side of the petrous temporal bone. Manifested as chronic headache, facial paralysis and a mild motor and static ataxia (right cerebellar hemisphere).
a, b) Preoperative MRI.
c, d) Peroperative views showing the diode laser being used in contact mode with a conical-tip shaped fibre (600 µm in diameter, emission power = 10 W cw) to fragment the tumour and induce effective haemostasis.

Neurosurgical applications

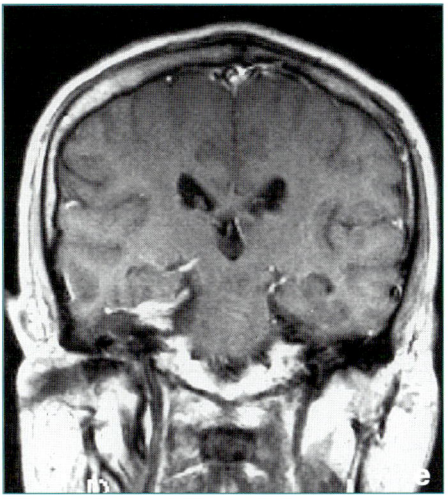
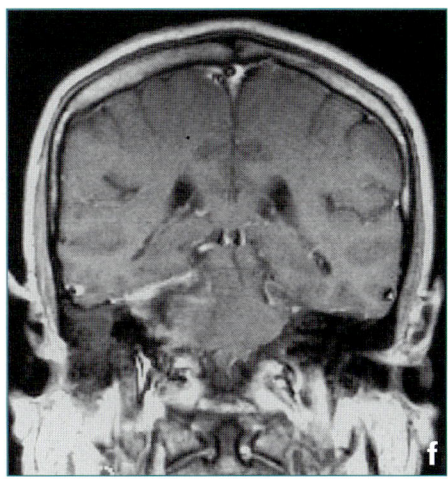

e, f) Postoperative MRI (performed 8 days after the operation) confirming that the tumour was completely excised. The brain stem and, in particular, the right cerebral peduncle, have returned to their normal positions. In clinical terms, two months after the operation, the patient was suffering some minor problems with swallowing, mild ataxia and some right facial paralysis which was regressing.

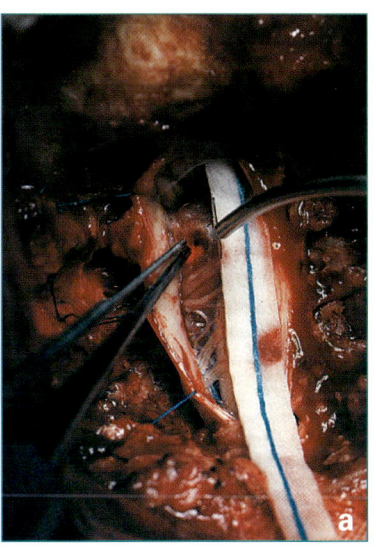
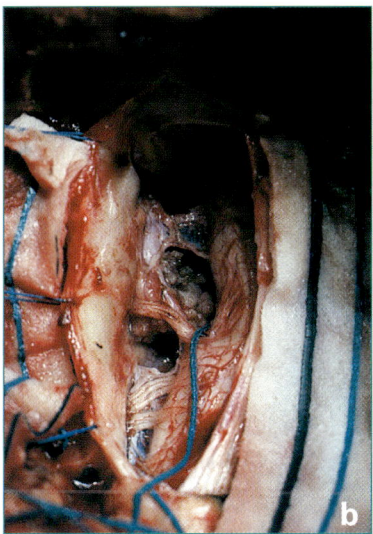
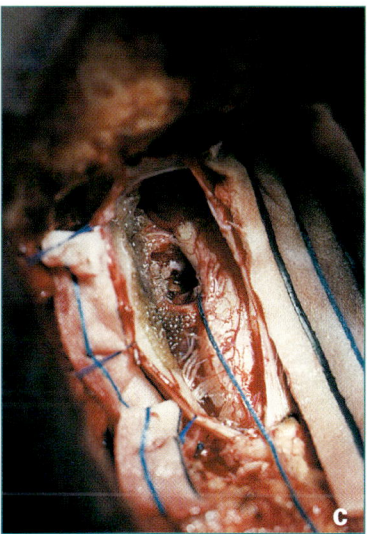

■ **Figure 17.** *Meningioma of the foramen magnum.*
A 43 year-old man who was admitted into the Department for asymmetric tetraparesis which was more marked on the right side.
a) On the opening of the dura mater, the meningioma can be clearly seen in front of the curtain formed by the superior cervical radicellae.
b, c) Removal of the tumour mainly by means of vaporisation using a diode laser operating in pulsed mode at an output power of 5 to 10 W. Higher power was used to vaporise tumour fragments near the insertion zone. Near the radicellae, power was decreased to 5 W. Given the very limited space between the radicellae, the CUSA could not be used because it was deemed to be too risky. Throughout the operation, the exposed spinal cord was protected from misdirected laser shots with moistened cotton pads.

operating time and in the amount of concomitant mechanical injury to neighbouring brain structures and intracranial nerves account for the improved success rates and the lower incidence of complications associated with such operations these days. In these delicate areas, the use of non-contact radiation is somewhat risky because of the possibility of diffusion; therefore we recommend using 600 or 1,000 µm conical shaped fibres. If a surgeon chooses to operate in non-contact mode with a micromanipulator or a very fine, long hand piece, the beam must be as highly focused as possible in order to make sure that the impact zone remains of sub-millimetre dimensions. Emission power should be kept low (5 to 10 W) and operation should be in pulsed mode to benefit from both the higher peak output power levels and the relaxation time between pulses.

In all cases, we use a 810 nm semiconductor laser in conjunction with the CUSA. In practice, the CUSA is only useful and practical if the tumour is relatively soft and it is when the tumour is too hard for such aspiration alone that the laser comes into its own because it can be used to fragment the mass while at the same time inhibiting bleeding. In this case, we tend to use a contact fibre to dissect out the fragments of the meningioma and coagulate the vessels at the cut surface – we use an output power of between 8 and 10 W cw. If the surgeon wishes to use a non-contact fibre to fragment the tumour, we recommend a 600 or 1,000 µm fibre with pulsed emission of the order of 15 W. In order to dissect or vaporise the tumour, the power can be raised to 20 to 25 W in pulsed mode. Haemostasis is achieved by putting the continuous beam out of focus (to a greater or lesser extent) by moving the hand piece away by a matter of a few millimetres or centimetres and reducing the emission power.

In our experience, using a 810 nm semiconductor laser (with or without CUSA) has reduced operating times and cut down on postoperative complications.

Figures 16, 17 and 18 show a few examples of the situations discussed in the preceding paragraphs.

■ Posterior cranial fossa schwannomas

Like meningiomas of the posterior cranial fossa, acoustic neuromas (or other types of cranial schwannoma) are **ideal candidates** for laser-assisted microsurgery. Again, we will not be discussing the problem of which approach to take to access the cerebellopontine angle but only which laser fibre should be chosen (*i.e.* diameter, shaped or not, etc.) and emission parameters.

As for most interventions, we prefer to use a hand piece rather than a micromanipulator which restricts the manoeuvrability of the beam. A CUSA machine has become almost essential for excising schwannomas with a diameter of 20 millimetres or over (grade 2 and above).

The tumour can be fragmented using a semiconductor laser with a 600 or 1,000 µm fibre in contact mode at an output power of 8 to

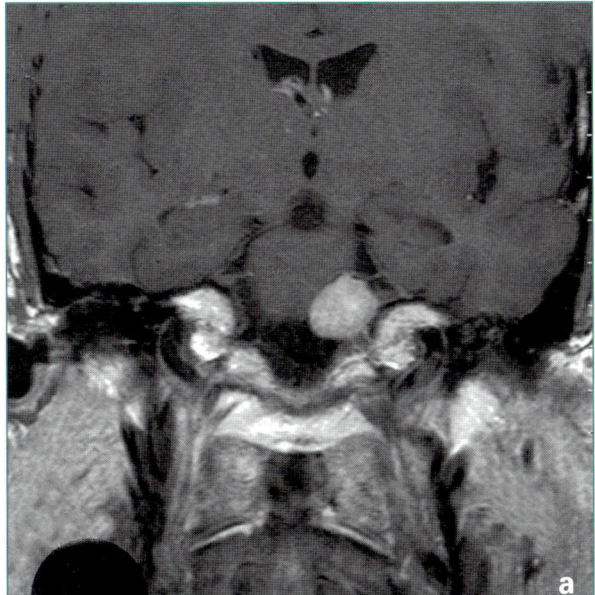

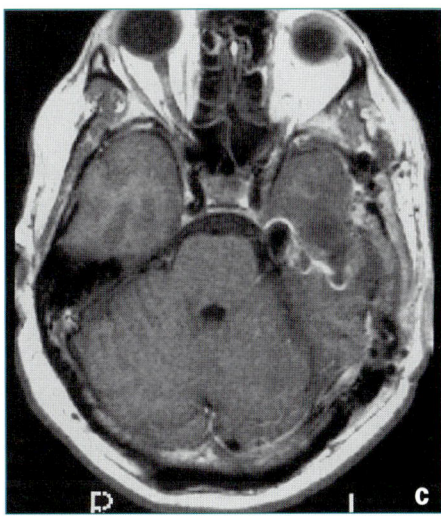

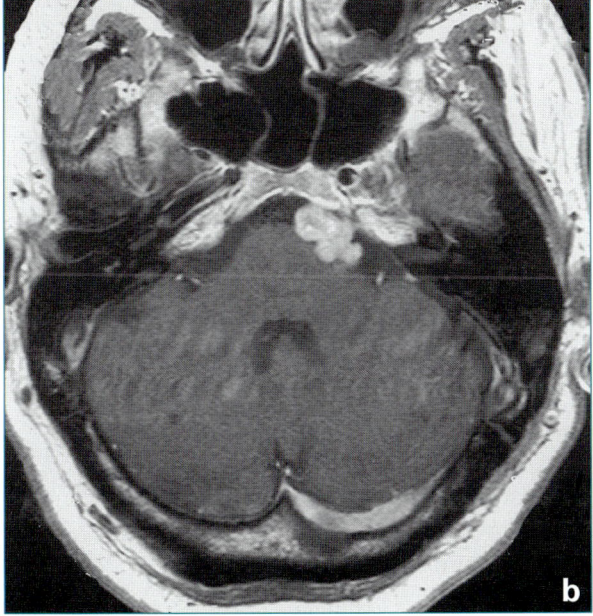

■ **Figure 18.** *A 50 year-old man with a left-petro-clival meningioma which manifested as left hemifacial hypoaesthesia (isolated involvement of the trigeminal nerve).*
a, b) Peroperative MRI.
c) Following a sub-temporal, sub-petrous approach, the 6-month follow-up MRI confirms that the tumour was completely removed.

10 W. Non-contact mode irradiation (at an emission power of 5 to 10 W cw) is useful for haemostasis within the tumour mass once it has been debulked by ultrasound cavitation aspiration but, given the proximity of the acoustic and facial nerves and the brain stem, it would seem wise to avoid non-contact operation if the capsule is being approached from either the anterior pole (touching the acoustic and facial nerves) or the middle (touching the side of the brain stem).

■ Brain stem tumours

Tumours involving the brain stem and the medulla oblongata are ideal candidates for treatment with a laser operating in continuous mode. A 600 or 1,000 µm shaped fibre can be used for making an incision in the brain stem tissue to gain access to a deeper lesion, be it a well defined tumour like a cavernous hemangioma or a diffuse one like a glioma *(figure 19)*. The great advantage of a diode laser with a contact fibre is that it can be used to both section and induce haemostasis in very delicate regions. If the tumour is a well defined one like an ependymoma or a cavernous hemangioma, a laser in contact mode can be used to define the plane of dissection between the tumour and the healthy tissue with as high a level of accuracy as possible while at the same time coagulating all the sectioned arterial and venous capillaries and stopping bleeding.

We recommend a low emission power of the order of 4 to 8 W cw, at which output level thermal diffusion around the shaped tip is virtually zero and the risk of damaging underlying structures very low.

■ Pituitary adenomas and craniopharyngiomas

• *Via* **an endonasal approach**. For a number of years now, we have not used a superior gingival trans-sphenoidal approach to gain access to the sella turcica but have been choosing the endonasal route, *i.e.* we pass the speculum and the other instruments between the mucosa and the right lateral side of the nasal septum. For some cases, we combine this procedure with endoscopy of the sellar cavity. For our part, we never use any type of laser radiation in this type of surgery but some surgeons use Nd-YAG lasers with fibre optic to induce haemostasis within the sella turcica. Nobody has yet suggested a role for diode lasers in the treatment of these kinds of tumour as this shows no particular benefit.

• *Via* **an intracranial approach**. When it comes to either invasive pituitary adenomas which require an intracranial approach, or cra-

Neurosurgical applications

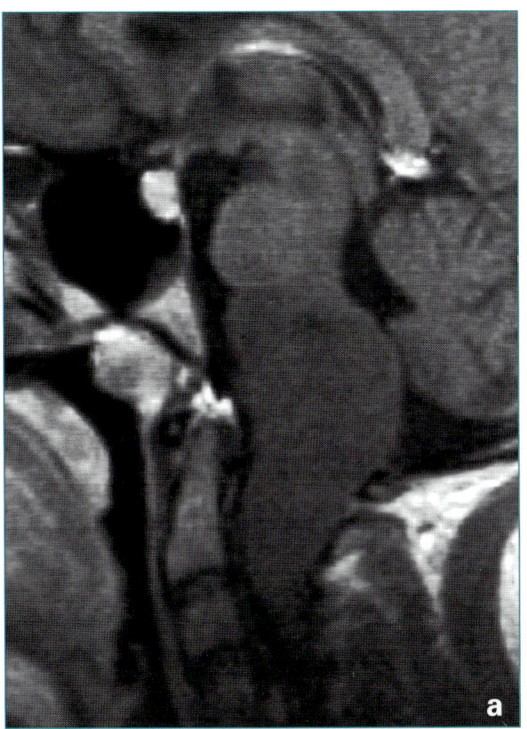
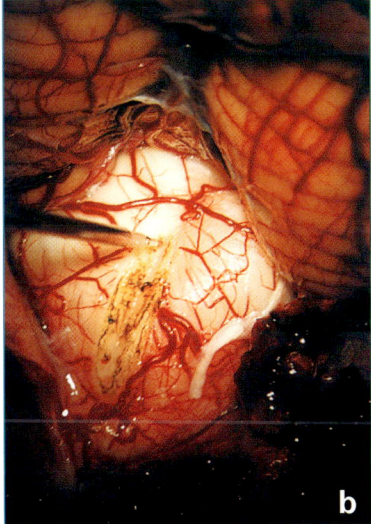
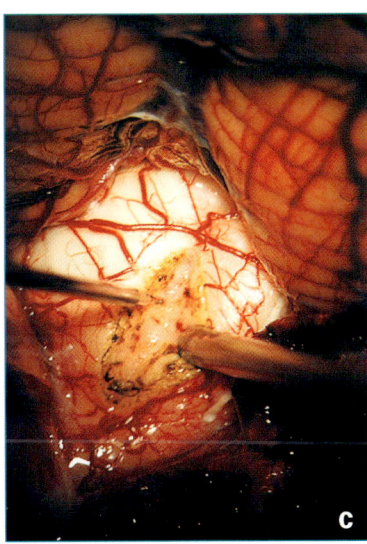

Figure 19. A 21 year-old woman with a medullo-pontine astrocytoma causing moderate, progressive tetraparesis and problems with swallowing.
a) T1 MRI after injection of gadolinium showing the swelling of the brain stem. The tumour is mainly infiltrating the medulla oblongata and the pons and pushing back the lower half of the IVth ventricle behind.
b, c) The aim of the intervention was to completely open the posterior cranial fossa and the foramen magnum in order to avoid inducing dangerous intracranial hypertension. The other purpose was to take a sizeable intramedullary biopsy for thorough pathological analysis before radiotherapy. A contact laser fibre (at 4 W cw) was used to make an incision in the posterior side of the medulla oblongata and provide access to the tumour without any bleeding.

niopharyngiomas which need to be completely or partially excised, our attitude is completely different. In this case, the problems are the same as with meningiomas located within the anterior base of the skull. The combination of a diode laser and the CUSA is ideal if such equipment is available in the operating theatre. Dissecting vascular structures and optic nerves is less risky with a shaped fibre (600 or 1,000 µm) and haemostasis within the tumour is more effectively achieved using a bare end non-contact fibre (8 to 15 W cw). In all cases, emission parameters must be carefully chosen and monitored when working near the third ventricle and the anterior columns of the fornix of cerebrum because even slight elevations in local temperature can entail post-operative loss of memory function of variable duration. Similarly, high power outputs should be avoided close to the lateral wall of the cavernous sinus because of the proximity of the oculomotor nerves. In our experience, we have observed postoperative oculomotor paralysis in two patients, both of which we attributed to over-heating of the region: fortunately, both patients recovered the lost function within a week.

■ Other tumours: metastases, gliomas, etc.

In our opinion, lasers are of very limited use or none at all in the surgical treatment of gliomas and astrocytomas insofar as conventional neurosurgical procedures are concerned. On the other hand, a laser guided by a robotic neuronavigation system can be useful in the vaporisation of small, deep tumours. This was proposed and first attempted over fifteen years ago by P. Kelly in the United States and he is still using CO_2 lasers for this type of procedure. We mentioned the value of combining lasers and the techniques of interventional navigation in the last chapter.

With respect to metastases, since such lesions are usually well limited and can be removed in one single piece, lasers are of little relevance.

■ Intraventricular endoscopic procedures

■ The intracranial use of endoscopes is not new but the development of as manoeuvrable a tool as the fibre optic-based diode laser massively increases the scope of the interventions which are possible without having to open up the skull. In general, we are proposing two types of procedure as amenable for laser-assisted endoscopy, namely the treatment of colloid cysts and the performing of ventriculocisternostomies.

■ Intraventricular tumours and colloid cysts

Although rare, a **colloid cyst in the third ventricle** represents an **ideal candidate** for laser-assisted endoscopic resection. Most rigid endoscopes have one or two working channels into which a fibre optic can be introduced. It should be noted that rigid endoscopes give a better image and are also more versatile than flexible models because the working channels are larger. During endoscopy, whether the medium be aqueous or air (after drainage of the CSF), a laser can be used to first coagulate the choroid plexuses which block the access of instruments and then to coagulate and shrink the cyst wall before perforation and vaporisation of the residue. This procedure involves the following steps: 1) coagulation and perforation of the cyst wall; 2) aspiration of the contents with a catheter or their removal using very fine forceps; 3) then the rest of the wall is coagulated and retracted so as to leave only its insertion zone. The kinds of laser which are suitable for this procedure are the 1.06 μm Nd-YAG type (for coagulating vessels in the wall), the 1.32 μm Nd-YAG type (for use in contact mode to coagulate the choroid plexus, perforate the cyst wall and then retract or vaporise it) or a diode laser which should be used in contact mode for perforating the wall and then in non-contact mode for coagulating the vessels. If there are fragments of carbonised tissue on the tip of the fibre, it should be cleaned before using in non-contact mode. This ensures efficient delivery of laser energy. All these lasers are used at emission powers of 4 to 10 W cw *(figure 20)*.

Other intraventricular tumours can be approached with an endoscope for taking biopsies, in which case a laser is useful for haemostasis of the surrounding tissue. Actual endoscopic removal of such tumours is rarely possible because of their dimensions and the restricted manoeuvrability of the instruments. Usually, a straight, stereotactically guided approach with microsurgical removal is the most effective modality.

■ Ventriculocisternostomy

Perforation of the basal third ventricle establishes communication between the ventricular cavities and the cisternae of the base of the skull and represents the treatment of choice for non-communicating hydrocephalus. Perforation can be accomplished by means of a mechanical instrument (an inflatable balloon or a coagulating pointed instrument) but using a laser gives a wider, less traumatic opening in the basal ventricle. The procedure which should be completed in as short a time as possible includes the following steps: 1) choice of a route for introducing the endoscope through the lateral ventricle, the interventricular foramen and the cavity of the third ventricle; 2) video-controlled introduction of the endoscope; 3) insertion of the laser fibre optic (usually a 400 μm bare end fibre) in the endoscope's working channel; 4) installation of multiple points of coagulation and perforation in the basal ventricle using the

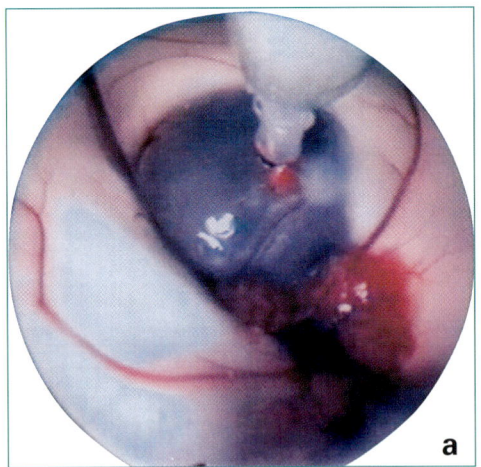
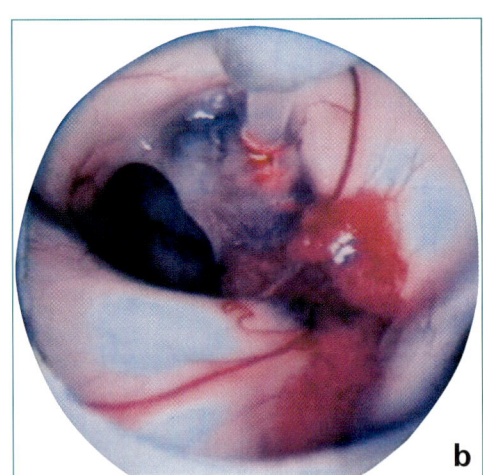
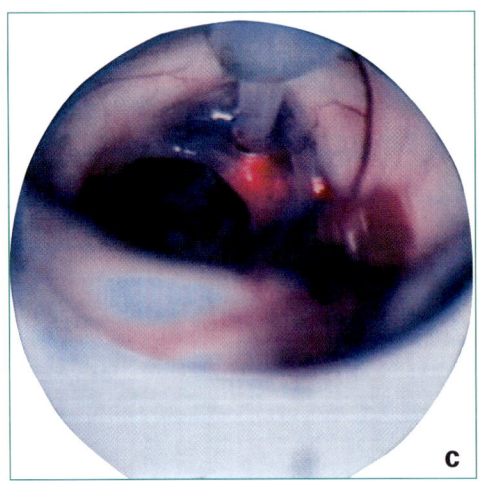
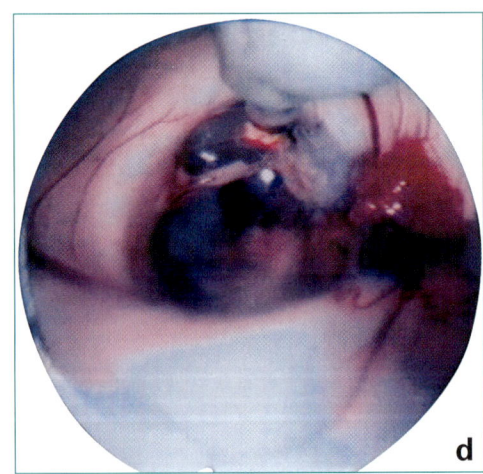

■ **Figure 20.** *Colloid cyst in the IIIrd ventricle. Treatment by laser stereo-endoscopy.*
a) An endoscopic view of the cyst at the beginning of the operation. The cyst is inserted in the left interventricular foramen. A series of laser shots (4 W cw) were fired to retract the cyst walls – this bleaches the capsule.
b, c) After incision of the capsule using a non-contact fibre at a distance of 1 to 2 mm (power = 6 W cw), the colloid material was aspirated and then the capsule was coagulated and almost completely retracted using endoscopic microforceps. Then the residual capsule material was coagulated and retracted with repeated laser shots.
d) At the end of the operation, the last bridges composed of fragments of the cyst's capsule are coagulated and sectioned with the diode laser fibre in non-contact mode at a power output of 6 W cw.
e) The foramen is completely free and gives access to the cavity of the third ventricle.

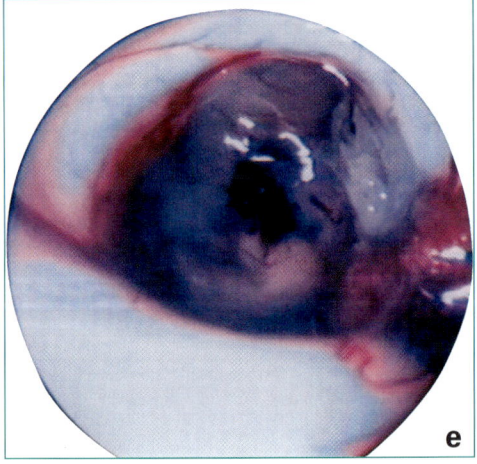

fibre in contact mode (the laser used could be a 1.32 μm Nd-YAG model at 6 to 8 W cw or a 810 nm diode model at 10 W with a carbonised fibre); 5) removal using very fine forceps of any fragments of the coagulated ventricular floor present in the perforation holes. The resultant hole should measure 4 x 4 mm, *i.e.* larger than most of the perforations which can be made by mechanical means which entails a reduced risk of secondary blockage *(figure 21)*.

■ Surgery for epilepsy

The idea of surgery for epilepsy (effectively drug-refractory, partial epilepsy) includes both interventions intended as curative – resection of a lesion or of the epileptogenic cortex – and palliative measures – corpuscallosotomy and hemispherectomy. As in general tumour surgery, lasers can be useful for the resection of structures or epileptogenic tumours. Diode lasers with a shaped fibre (600 or 1,000 μm in diameter with a conical 300 μm tip) in contact mode are especially useful for coagulating and cutting gyri in the epileptogenic zone which are often firmer than non-pathological gyri. Resection of the hippocampus projecting in the temporal horn of lateral ventricle and almost always involved in cases of temporal epilepsy is easier with the diode laser in contact mode.

Otherwise, although still in the research stage, our team has proposed an experimental model in which a network of cortical photo-induced lesions might represent a surgical alternative to cortical resection, especially if the epileptogenic zone coincides with a functionally important region of the brain.

■ Intraspinal tumours

■ The most suitable intraspinal tumours for diode laser-assisted surgery are meningiomas, schwannomas, lipomas of the cauda equina and, perhaps most of all, intramedullary tumours.

■ Extradural and/or intradural tumours

Meningiomas

The same advantages and disadvantages apply to laser treatment of this type of intraspinal tumour as previously discussed in the context of the intracranial, supratentorial and subtentorial forms.

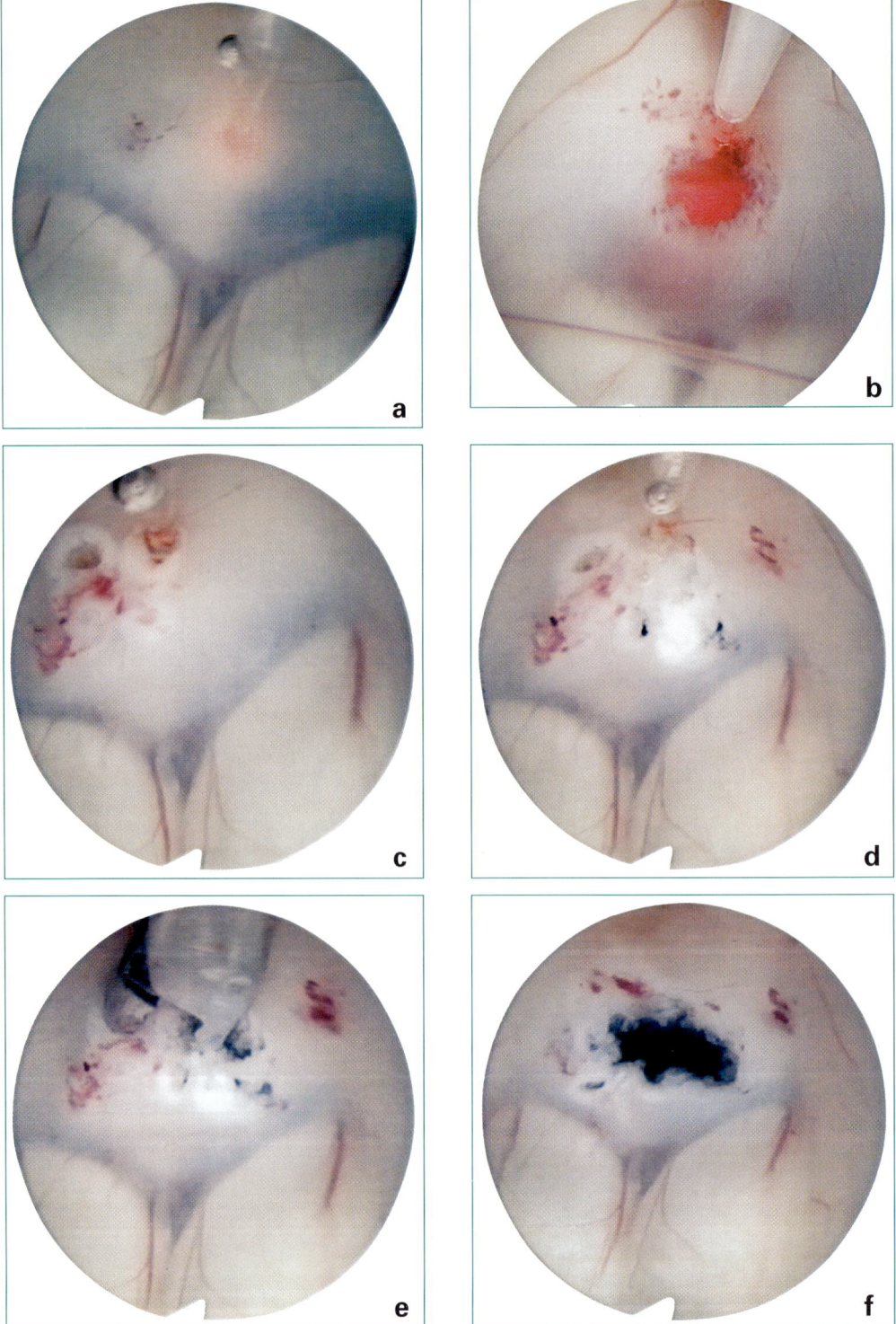

■ **Figure 21.** *Ventriculocysternostomy. a) Endoscopic view of the basal third ventricle: the opening should be made in front of the mamillary bodies (the white structures in the lower part of the view). The laser fibre (bare end, 400 μm fibre) is visible in contact with the basal ventricle. b) A one second laser shot at 5 W cw induces contact photocoagulation and makes a perforation with the same diameter as the fibre. c, d) Repeated laser shots to form a network across the surface to be covered: between the perforations, the bridging basal ventricle tissue is coagulated by adjacent shots. e) The fragments of coagulated tissue between the perforations are removed using microforceps. f) The appearance of the opening at the end of the operation: adjacent nervous structures are completely untouched and the dimensions of the opening are 4 × 3 mm.*

After appropriately opening the vertebral canal by laminectomy according to the position of the tumour (preaxial, anterolateral, lateral or posterior), a diode laser can be used as a first step to heat the tumour and induce its retraction. This should be performed with a relatively high intensity but out-of-focus beam (around 10 to 15 W cw). Since intraspinal meningiomas usually occur in an anterolateral position, the denticulate ligament will often have to be sectioned to gain access to the lesion. This can be accomplished using a diode laser in non-contact mode with a focused beam (10 to 15 W in pulsed mode), or better still with a shaped fibre. Of course, the ligament can also be cut using microscissors. Retraction of the meningioma facilitates release of the arachnoidea matter which separates it from the spinal cord. After incision into the capsule in either contact or non-contact mode, the meningioma can be fragmented with a contact fibre and/or the CUSA. Throughout all laser-mediated sectioning and coagulation exercises, it is essential to make sure that all spinal cord tissue and radicellae are thoroughly protected by cotton pads. If all or part of the tumour is in front of the medulla, it can be vaporised and/or coagulated with the laser beam incident at an oblique angle – this is made possible by the small size of today's hand pieces which can be both shaped relatively easily and can also be adapted to give to the radiation the exact desired angle. At the end of the intervention, the insertion zone of the tumour should be charred using the diode laser in non-contact mode (10 to 15 W in pulsed mode).

Intraspinal schwannomas

The problems with schwannomas are similar to those encountered with meningiomas. Insofar as schwannomas are closely associated with the roots and radicellae, we prefer to use the laser in contact mode. A 600 µm shaped fibre can be used to: accurately dissect out the tumour without damaging any nerve fibres; progressively fragment the schwannoma while at the same time inducing haemostasis of the cut surface. However, in some cases, bipolar coagulation might be more effective than the laser or it might be best to use both tools at the same time. Similarly, for reducing the tumour, CUSA can and should be used together with the laser and the microscissors.

Intraspinal lipomas *(figure 22)*

These are particularly amenable to diode laser treatment, especially the terminal and posterior forms of lipoma of the cone of the spinal cord and of the cauda equina. In the former case, sub-dural lipomas can be easily separated from the roots of the cauda equina and can be sectioned using either conventional techniques (microscissors and bipolar coagulation) or a diode laser; this is most simply

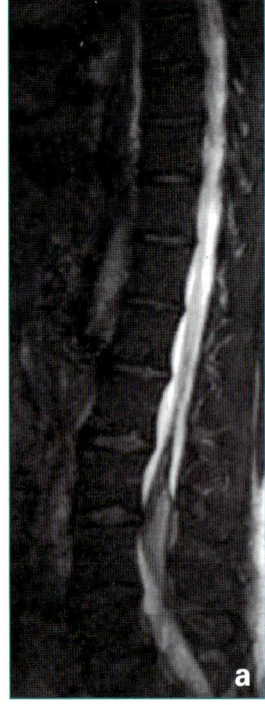
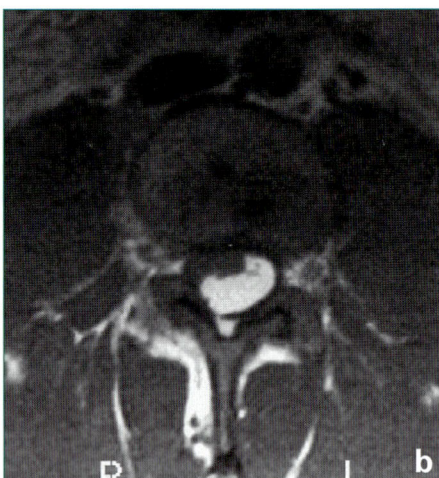

■ **Figure 22.** *Lipoma of the equina cauda. A 29 year-old patient who had been suffering from mild genito-urinary problems for the previous three months.
a) Sagittal MRI in echo with a T2 gradient showing the lipoma extending from the lower edge of L2 to the upper edge of L5.
b) Axial MRI slice.*

accomplished using a 600 μm conical shaped fibre with precautions to avoid haemorrhagic suffusion. Posterior forms present more problems because such lipomas are often very closely associated with the roots which can be fairly deeply embedded within it. Hitherto, exeresis of the lipoma and dissection of the roots was performed using conventional instruments but, over the last ten years, these operations have been made much easier by the availability of the CUSA which can be used to progressively evacuate the lipoma with a minimum of traction force exerted on the roots and the terminal cone of the spinal cord. More recently still, the application of diode lasers in contact mode has allowed very accurate dissection of the adipose lobules which are in direct contact with the nerve roots with simultaneous efficient haemostasis. The combination of two different tools, the CUSA and the diode laser, has transformed such surgery of bulky lipomas by reducing the risk of mechanical traction force damaging nearby nervous structures (radicellae, the terminal cone of the spinal cord and the medulla). Radiation from a non-contact fibre seems to us less easy to control in terms of unwanted heating because the roots are often stuck together and, at the same time, buried in the adipose lobules.

Neurosurgical applications

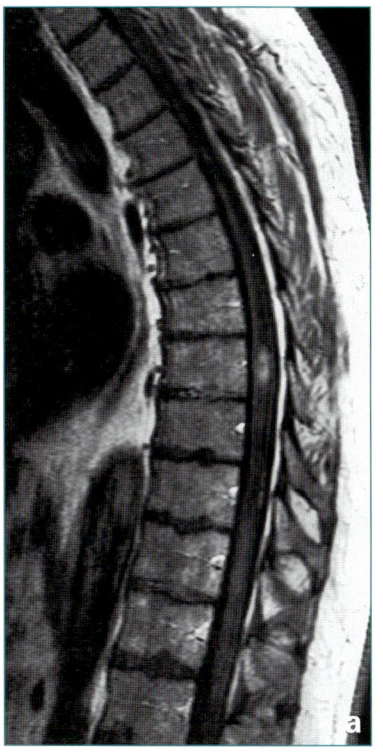
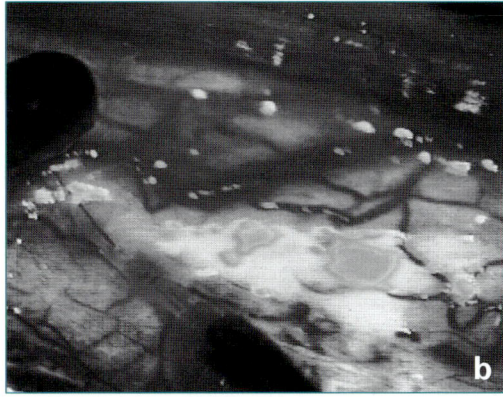
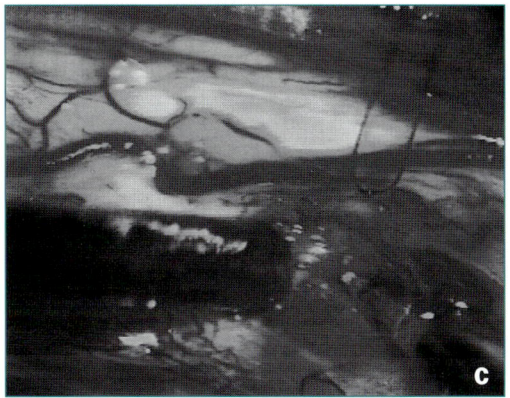
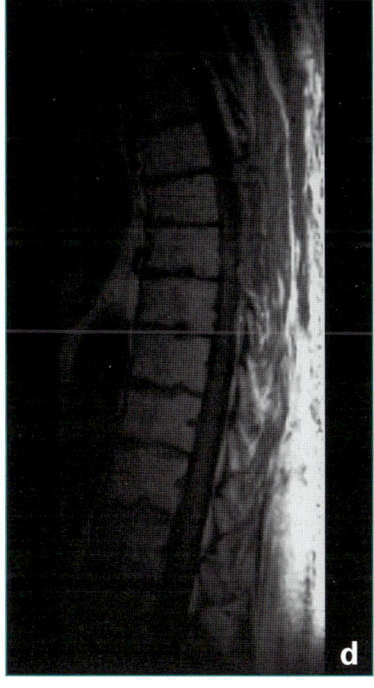

■ **Figure 23.** *Intramedullary thoracic ependymoma (T8) causing slowly progressive paraparesis in a 52 year-old man.*
a) Preoperative MRI; T1 sagittal slice: the tumour is opposite the 8th dorsal vertebra and appears hyperintense and relatively homogenous.
b) Peroperative view: myelotomy performed using a contact fibre (power = 4 W cw).
c) Peroperative view: dissection and drainage of the tumour performed using a power output of 5 to 6 W cw.
d) The 6-month follow-up MRI after complementary radiotherapy shows that the tumour was completely excised in the operation. Two years after the intervention, the patient was walking almost normally.

■ Diode lasers in neurosurgery

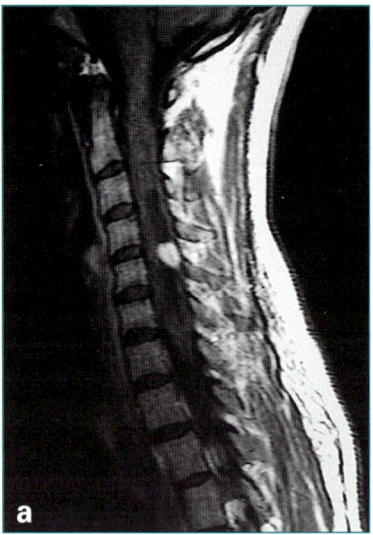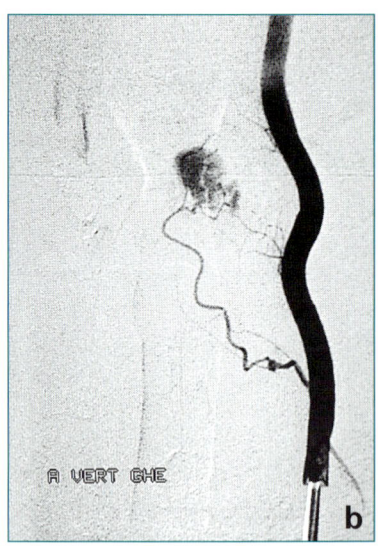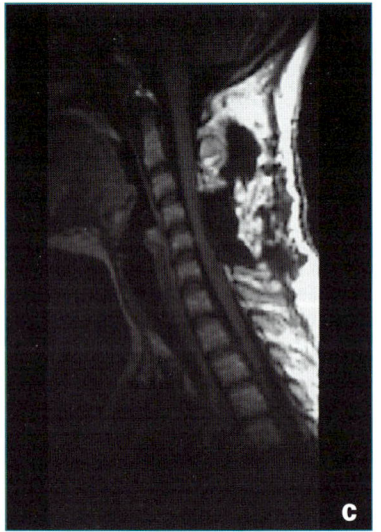

■ **Figure 24.** *Intramedullary cervical (C4-C5) hemangioblastoma in a 34 year-old woman causing asymmetric tetraparesis which was more marked on the right side.*
a) MRI showing the hyperintense hemangioma.
b) Left vertebral angiography allowing injection of the tumour.
c) The 10-month follow-up MRI confirms that intraspinal morphology has returned to normal.
Removal of the tumour in one piece was followed by complete neurological recovery. By 12 months after the operation, the only remaining problems were some pyramidal symptoms affecting the lower limbs and mild hypoaesthesia in the left leg.

■ **Intramedullary tumours**

There are two main reasons for using diode lasers in surgery for intramedullary tumours: firstly for performing myelotomy and secondly to help excise the intra-axial lesion itself. We recommend that, for tumours in this region, the laser should only be used in contact mode with a 600 or 1,000 µm conical shaped fibre.

Using a diode laser in contact mode for myelotomy guarantees haemostasis of the cut surfaces at the same time as the incision is made to access the medulla. For this purpose, we use a 600 µm conical shaped fibre with an output power of 5 ± 1 W. The advantage of using a laser in contact mode compared with bipolar electrocoagulation is the fact that there is no diffusion of heat which is restricted to the very tip of the shaped fibre – this is why the beam simultaneously coagulates and sections the tissue. Using a diode laser in contact mode therefore precludes haemorrhagic suffusion around the myelotomy and is, in our opinion, **unequalled for this type of procedure**.

Insofar as **exeresis of the tumour** is concerned, this should be performed using the CUSA, whatever the nature of the tumour, be it an ependymoma or a glial lesion *(figure 23)*. However, a shaped fibre can be useful and effective in the fragmentation of the tumour. This is mainly because it induces haemostasis of the intratumoural capillaries which are exposed by the CUSA. In the special case of intramedullary hemangiomas, a semiconductor diode laser used with a contact fibre can of course be used to perform the myelotomy and also for defining the plane of dissection and excising the lesion without causing any intraspinal bleeding *(figure 24)*. These represent ideal circumstances for using a diode laser in contact mode.

Future perspectives

Future perspectives for the use of lasers in medicine are closely associated with the development of new minimally invasive operating techniques. So far in this context, semiconductor diode lasers have proven one of the most promising of the tools already in existence.

■ Miniaturisation

Although diodes have already meant huge reductions in size in the lasers used for medical applications, the process of miniaturisation is certainly going to accelerate in the years to come. Tomorrow's lasers will be smaller, more specific, computer-controlled and designed to be linked to other diagnostic and imaging devices.

■ "Smart" lasers and tunable pocket lasers

The true revolution to come in terms of laser technology will be the development of highly versatile lasers which will be able to emit a range of different types of beam, *e.g.* by doubling or tripling the basic wavelength. Cybernetic-type control systems applied to such multifunctional lasers will make them into "smart" machines which will be able to select the appropriate wavelength according to the circumstances, *e.g.* is heat needed or is the procedure one of simple photoablation? The choice of which wavelength to emit will not depend only on the kind of effect sought vis-à-vis the target tissue but also on specific characteristics of that tissue which the machine will be able to analyse and take into account. Specific markers for labelling tissues will help the machine recognise different tissue types and determine their properties – existing markers like HPD (hematoporphyrin derivatives) and DHE are only precursors for a wide range of such specific markers which are in the process of development in immunohistochemical research laboratories.

■ Robotisation

The future will also see the development of increasingly sophisticated robotic laser guidance systems parallel to those integrated into the kind of computer-assisted imaging systems and peroperative neuronavigation equipment already being widely installed in neurosurgery operating theatres. We already mentioned in Chapter 6 the great contribution being made by the application of the techniques of interventional navigation and it is certain that the linking of these techniques with an instrument-guiding robotic system which could entirely or partially control the movements involved in stereotactic removal procedures would enormously facilitate this kind of operation, *e.g.* by directing a laser beam with pinpoint accuracy.

■ "Laser" fibres

With respect to semiconductor diode lasers, the innovation which is due to appear on the market next involves special laser fibres, the development of which is currently underway. The special features of these fibres are due to the fact that they are doped with a Rare Earth metal like neodymium which results in the emission of radiation at 1.06 μm when coupled to a diode laser. Power of up to about 15 W can be put out at the tip of the fibre. Other doping substances are being investigated including simultaneous doping with Er^{3+} and Yb^{3+} which gives a fibre which produces radiation at 1.55 μm. A fibre doped with Tm^{3+} emits in the 2.0 μm spectral band. Obviously, such fibres will considerably extend the potential of high power diode lasers, especially given that multifibre connectors are being developed to make it possible to switch from one wavelength to another as the need arises.

■ Ultrafast lasers

The use of the non-thermal effects of laser radiation in neurosurgery is still at the experimental stage although tissue photoablation is already being used in both ophthalmology (corneal resurfacing) and dental surgery (dental cavitation). Photoablation by fast thermal explosion which induces plasma-mediated volatilisation of tissue (a non-thermal mechanism) has enormous potential as does electromechanical tissue disruption at the molecular level. Such techniques would facilitate the removal of tumours and reduce the damage associated with such procedures in certain regions of the body, *e.g.* intraventricular tumours, tumours of the cerebellopontine angle or those in contact with the brain stem, in fact in any situation where surgical access is confined and any kind of mechanical stress has to be avoided.

■ Lasers in diagnosis

The diagnostic application of lasers and other sources of monochromatic light in a range of different disciplines – dermatology, urology, ophthalmology, pneumology and gastroenterology – represents a fast-growing field. Currently, fluorescent imaging techniques, optical coherence tomography and elastic diffusion spectroscopy are all biophotonic imaging techniques which are being actively investigated. The special difficulties associated with the nervous system mainly derive from its opacity and its protection, which constitutes an obstacle to the propagation of photons and analysis of the tissue. New techniques are being called upon. In the future, the spectral profile of healthy and diseased tissue – **their so-called optical biopsy** – could be a powerful, non-invasive diagnostic tool in neurology as in other disciplines. During surgical operations, such techniques could soon become indispensable for checking whether a tumour has been completely excised or not.

Bibliography

- Abernathey CD, Davis DH, Kelly PJ. Treatment of colloid cyst of the third ventricle by stereotaxic microsurgery. *J Neurosurg* 1989; 70: 525-529.
- Amin Z, Buonaccorsi G, Mills T, Harries S, Lees WR, Bown SG. Interstitial laser photocoagulation: evaluation of a 1320 Nd-YAG and an 805 nm diode laser: the significance of charring and the value of pre-charring the fibre tip. *Lasers Med Sci* 1993; 8: 113-120.
- Amin Z. Diode lasers: experimental and clinical review. *Lasers Med Sci* 1995; 10: 157-163.
- Auer LM, Holzer P, Ascher PW, Heppner F. Endoscopic neurosurgery. *Acta Neurochirurgica* 1988; 90: 1-14.
- Bartal AD, Heilbron VD, Avram J. Carbon dioxide laser of basal meningiomas. *Surg Neurol* 1982; 17: 90-95.
- Bayly IG, Karth VB, Stevence WH. The absorption spectra of liquid phase H_2O, HDO and D_{20} from 0.7 µm to 10 µm. *Infr Phys* 1963; 3: 211-223.
- Beck OJ. The use of the Nd-YAG and the CO_2 laser in neurosurgery. *Neurosurg Rev* 1980; 3: 261-266.
- Blanc D, Colles MJ. Transmission measurements on various samples between 1,064 nm and 2,000 nm. *Lasers Med Sci* 1990; 5: 71-75.
- Boulnois JL. Photophysical process in recent medical laser development. *Lasers Med Sci* 1986; 1: 47-66.
- Brunetaud JM, Chavoin JP, Gaillot-Mangin J, Godart B, Lecarpentier Y, Laffitte F, Mordon S, Roux FX, Sultan R. *Encyclopédie des Lasers en Médecine et en Chirurgie. Bases physiques et principes fondamentaux.* Piccin Ed., Padoue, Italy, 1995: 499.
- Brunetaud JM, Mordon S. L'Avenir des Lasers Médicaux. *Neurochirurgie* 1992; 38: 248-251.
- Craford MG. Recent developments in LED technology. *IEEE Trans Elect Dev* 1977; ED-24: 935.
- Decq P, Le Guerinel C, Brugières P, Djindjian M, Silva D, Kéravel Y, Melon E, Nguyen JP. Endoscopic management of colloid cysts. Clinical study. *Neurosurgery* 1998; 42: 1288-1296.
- Desgeorges M, Sterkers O, Ducolombier A, Pernot P et col. La microchirurgie au laser des méningiomes. Analyse d'une série consécutive de 164 opérés avec différents lasers. *Neurochirurgie* 1992; 38: 217-225.
- Desgeorges M, Sterkers O, Poncet JL, Rey A, Sterkers JM. Chirurgie des Méningiomes de la partie postérieure de la Base du Crâne. 135 cas. Choix de la Voie d'abord et Résultats. *Neurochirurgie* 1995; 4: 265-294.

- Devaux B, Lamarche M, Fallet-Bianco C, Olive L, Catala I, Roux FX. Photolésions corticales multiples et foyer épileptogène à la pénicilline. *Neurochirurgie* 1996; 42: 153-161.
- Devaux B, Roux FX. Experimental and Clinical Standards, and Evolution of Lasers in Neurosurgery. *Acta Neurochirurgica* 1996; 138: 1135-1147.
- Devaux B, Roux FX, Nataf F, Turak B, Cioloca C. High power Diode Laser in Neurosurgery. Clinical Experience in 30 cases. *Surg Neurol* 1998; 50: 33-40.
- Dilkes MG, Cameron I, Quinn SJ, Kenyon GS. Preliminary experience with an 810 nm wavelength diode laser in ENT surgery. *Lasers Med Sci* 1994; 9: 261-264.
- Edwards MS, Boggan JE, Fuller TA. The laser in neurological surgery. *J Neurosurg* 1983; 59: 555-566.
- Eggert HR, Blazek V. Optical properties of human brain tissue, meninges and brain tumors in the spectral range of 200 to 900 nm. *Neurosurgery* 1987; 21: 459-464.
- Endriz JG, Vakili M, Browder GS. High-power diode-laser arrays. *IEEE J Quant Elect* 1992; 28: 952-965.
- Fernie DP, Mannonen I, Raven T. Small core fiber coupled 60 W laser diode. *SPIE Proceedings* 1995; 2396: 178-181.
- Frank F. Biophysical basis and technical requisites for the use of Nd-YAG laser in neurosurgery. *Neurosurg Rev* 1984; 7: 145-150.
- Geusic JE, Marcos HM, Van Uitert JG. Laser oscillations in Nd-doped yttrium aluminium, yttrium gallium and yttrium gadolinium garnets. *Appl Phys Lett* 1964; 4: 182-184.
- Godlewski G, Frapier JM, De Balmann B, Mouzayek H et col. Diode laser and microvascular carotid anastomosis: a preliminary study. *Lasers Med Sci* 1993; 8: 33-38.
- Greenwell TJ, Wyman A, Rogers K. Potentiation of laser-tissue interactions of the 805 nm laser with indocyanine green. *Lasers Med Sci* 1993; 8: 283-287.
- Griffith HB. Endoneurosurgery: endoscopic intracranial surgery. *Advances and Technical Standards in Neurosurgery,* vol.14, Springer-Verlag, Wien, New York, 1986: 2-24.
- Hebeda KM, Menovski T, Beek JF, Wolbers JG, Van Gemert JF. *Neurosurgery* 1994; 35: 720-724.
- Jacques S, Thomsen S, Schwartz J, Motamedi M, Rastegar S, Mannonen I. Comparing tissue optics and coagulation for a diode laser (805 nm) *versus* the Nd-YAG laser (1,064 nm). *Lasers Surg Med* 1992; 4 (suppl.): abst. 9.
- Jacques SL, Rastegar S, Motamedi M, Thomsen SL, Schwartz J, Torres J, Mannonen I. Liver photocoagulation with diode laser (805 nm) *vs* Nd-YAG laser (1,064 nm). *SPIE*, vol. 1646 Laser-tissue interaction III, 1992: 107-117.
- Jain KK. *Handbook of laser surgery*. Springfield Ill., Charles C. Thomas, 1983: 147 pp.
- Jain KK. Complications of the use of the Nd-YAG laser in neurosurgery. *Neurosurgery* 1985; 16: 759-762.
- Javan A, Bennett WR, Herriot DR. Population inversion and continuous optical laser oscillation in a gas discharge containing a He-Ne mixture. *Phys Rev Lett* 1961; 6: 106.
- Judy MM, Matthews JL, Aronoff BL, Hults DF. Soft tissue studies with 805 nm diode laser radiation: thermal effects with contact tips and comparison with effects of 1,064 nm Nd-YAG laser radiation. *Lasers Surg Med* 1993; 13: 528-536.
- Kaplan I, Aravot O, Giler S *et al.* Basic science. The clinical potential of Holmium laser. *Laser Med Surg* 1987; 3: 207-209.
- Kelly PJ, Alker GJ Jr. A stereotactic approach to deep seated CNS neoplasms using the carbon dioxide laser. *Surg Neurol* 1981; 15: 331-334.

- Kelly PJ, Alker GJ Jr, Goerss SJ. Computer assisted sterotactic laser microsurgery for the treatment of intracranial neoplasms. *Neurosurgery* 1982; 10: 324-331.

- Kelly PJ, Alker GJ Jr, Kall B, Goerss SJ. Precision resection of intra-axial CNS lesions by CT-based stereotactic craniotomy and computer monitored CO_2 laser. *Acta Neurochirurgica* 1983; 68: 1-9.

- Kelly PJ, Regli L, Al-Rodhan. Le laser au dioxide de carbone et la crâniotomie stéréotaxique. *Neurochirurgie* 1992; 38: 208-216.

- Lajat Y, Patrice T, Nomballais F, Nogues B, Resche F. Effects of 1.06 µm wavelength laser radiation applied stereotactically to brain tissue. *Laser Med Surg* 1987; 3: 45-51.

- Lerner EJ. Lasers diodes and LEDs light optoelectronic devices. *Laser Focus World* 1997; February: 109-117.

- Lerner EJ. Diode-laser wavelengths shift deeper into the infrared. *Laser Focus World* 1998; February: 95-102.

- Lerner EJ. Diode Lasers offer efficiency and reliability. *Laser Focus World* 1998; March: 93-98.

- McHugh JD, Marshall J, Ffytche TJ, Hamilton AM, Raven A, Keeler CR. Initial clinical experience using a diode laser in the treatment of retinal vascular disease. *Eye* 1989; 3: 516-527.

- Maiman TH. Stimulated optical radiation in ruby lasers. *Nature* 1960; 187: 493.

- Malcom GPA, Ferguson AI. Diode-pumped solid-state lasers. *Contem Phys* 1991; 32: 305-319.

- Manni J. Surgical diode lasers. *J Clinical Laser Med Surg* 1992; 10 (5): 377-380.

- Martiniuk R, Bauer JA, McKean JD, Tulip J, Mielke B. New long wavelength Nd-YAG laser at 1.44 µm: effect on brain. *J Neurosurg* 1989; 70: 249-256.

- Merienne L, Leriche B, Roux FX, Devaux B. Utilisation du Laser Nd-YAG en Endoscopie Intra-crânienne. Expérience préliminaire en Stéréotaxie. *Neurochirurgie* 1992; 38: 245-247.

- Minelly JD, Taylor ER, Jedrzejewski KP, Wang J, Payne DN. Laser diode pumped Nd^{3+} fibre laser with output power > 1 watt. *Proc CLEO*, Anaheim CA, 1992, CWE6.

- Minelly JD, Laming RI, Townsend JE, Barnes WL, Taylor ER, Jedrzejewski KP, Payne DN. High-gain amplifier tandem-pumped with a 3 W multistripe diode. *Proc OFC*, San Jose CA, 1992, TuG2.

- Minelly JD, Barnes WL, Laming RI, Morkel PR, Townsend JE, Grubb SG, Payne DN. Diode array pumping of Er^{3+} Yb^{3+} co-doped fiber lasers and amplifiers. *IEEE Photonics Tech Lett* 1993; 5, 4: 301-303.

- Mordon S, Roux FX, Mondragon S, Fallet-Bianco C, Sahafi F, Brunetaud JM. A comparative study of coagulation effects on the cortex of the rat using Nd-Yag (1.32 µm), Nd-YAG (1.06 µm) and CO_2 lasers. *Lasers Med Sci* 1990; 5: 293-296.

- Mordon S, Brunetaud JM. Bases physiques des applications thérapeutiques des lasers. *Neurochirurgie* 1992; 38: 203-207.

- Müller G, Dörschel K, Kar H. Biophysics of the photoablation process. *Lasers Med Sci* 1991; 6: 241-254.

- Patel CKN. Continuous wave laser action on vibrational-rotational transitions of CO_2. *Phys Rev A* 1964; 136: 1187-1193.

- Patterson MS, Wilson BC, Wyman DR. The propagation of optical radiation in tissue, 1. Models of radiation transport and their application. *Lasers Med Sci* 1991; 6: 155-168.

- Patterson MS, Wilson BC, Wyman DR. The propagation of optical radiation in tissue, 2. Optical properties of tissues and resulting fluence distributions. *Lasers Med Sci* 1991; 6: 379-390.

- Peyman GA, Cruz SA, Ruiz-Lapuente C. Contact diode laser application through a fiberoptic cutting tip. *Lasers Surg Med* 1991; 11: 347-350.
- Pierre-Kahn A, Zerah M, Renier D et col. Lipomes malformatifs intra-rachidiens. La chirurgie. *Neurochirurgie* 1995; 41 (suppl. 1): 88-99.
- Rastegar S, Jacques SL, Motamedi M, Kim BM. Theoretical analysis of equivalency of high-power diode laser (810 nm) and Nd-YAG (1,064 nm) for coagulation of tissue: predictions for prostate coagulation. *SPIE*, vol 1646 Laser tissue interaction III, 1992: 150-160.
- Raven A, Mannonen I, Fernie D. 25 watts high power diode lasers for surgical applications. *Lasers Surg Med* 1992; 4 (suppl.): abstr. 161.
- Raven T, Mannonen I, Fernie D. High power diode lasers and their surgical applications. *SPIE Proceedings* 1993; 1892: 12-16.
- Ripley PM. The physics of Diode Lasers. *Lasers Med Sci* 1996; 11: 71-78.
- Rouge D, Chavoin JP, Costagliola M, Arbus L. Évolution de la jurisprudence en matière de contrat médical en chirugie esthétique. *Ann Chir Plast Esth* 1990; 35 (4): 297-303.
- Roux FX. Le laser CO_2 neurochirurgical. Éd. Maloine, Paris 1986: p. 92.
- Roux FX, Mordon S, Mondragon S, Sahafi F, Fallet-Bianco C, Brunetaud JM. Le laser Nd-YAG 1,320 μm. Étude expérimentale d'une nouvelle longueur d'onde adaptée à la neurochirurgie. *Neurochirurgie* 1989; 35: 152-157.
- Roux FX, Merienne L, Cioloca C, Devaux B, Chodkiewicz JP. Neurosurgical Lasers for Tumour Removal. *Lasers Med Sci* 1990; 5: 241-244.
- Roux FX, Merienne L, Devaux B, Leriche B, Cioloca C. Les lasers YAG en neurochirurgie. *Neurochirurgie* 1992; 38: 229-234.
- Saunders ML, Young HG, Becker DP et al. The use of the laser in neurological surgery. *Surg Neurol* 1980; 14: 1-10.
- Sculpher MJ. A preliminary economic evaluation of the diode laser in ophthalmology. *Lasers Med Sci* 1993; 8: 163-169.
- Sterenborg HJ, Van Gemert MJ, Kamphorst W, Wolbers JG, Hogervorst W. The spectral dependance of the optical properties of the human brain. *Lasers Med Sci* 1989; 4: 221-227.
- Svaasand LO, Ellingsen R. Optical properties of human brain. *Photochem Photobiol* 1983; 38: 293-299.
- Takeuchi J, Handa H, Taki W, Yamagami T. The Nd-Yag laser in neurosurgical surgery. *Surg Neurol* 1982; 18: 140-142.
- Takizawa T, Yamakazi I. Laser surgery of basal, orbital and ventricular meningiomas which are difficult to extirpate by conventional methods. *Neuro Med Chir (Tokyo)* 1980; 20: 719-737.
- Tew JM, Tobler WD. The laser: history, biophysics and neurosurgical applications. *Clin Neurosurg,* Williams Wilkins ed., Baltimore, Chicago, Ill., 1983; 31: 506-549.
- Van Best JA, Schuitmaker HJ, Dubbelman TM, Van der Poel CJ, Fakkel J. Near infrared diode laser for photodynamic tumour therapy using bacteriochlorin *a. Lasers Med Sci* 1993; 8: 157-162.
- Wharen RE, Anderson RE, Scheithauer B, Sundt TM. The Nd-YAG laser in neurosurgery: dose related biological response of neural tissue. *J Neurosurg* 1984; 60: 531-539.
- Wyman A, Duffy S, Sweetland HM, Sharp F, Rogers K. Preliminary evaluation of a new high power diode laser. *Lasers Surg Med* 1992; 12: 506-509.
- Wyman A. Laser-tissue interactions of diode laser at 805 nm. *Lasers Surg Med* 1992; 4 (suppl.): 85.

References relevant to other types of surgery

- Bhatta KM. Urological applications with a 50 W diode laser. *Medical Laser Buyers Guide* 1995: 108-109.
- Brancato R, Pratesi R. Applications of diode laser in ophthalmology. *Lasers Ophthalmol* 1987; 1: 119-129.
- Brancato R, Carassa R, Trabucchi G. Diode laser compared with argon laser for trabeculoplasty. *Am J Ophthalmol* 1991; 112: 50-55.
- Dilkes MG, Cameron I, Quinn SJ, Kenyon GS. Preliminary experience with an 810 nm wavelength diode laser in ENT surgery. *Lasers Med Sci* 1994; 9: 261-264.
- Jacques SL, Rastegar S, Motamedi M. Liver photocoagulation with diode laser (805 nm) vs Nd-YAG laser (1,064 nm). *SPIE Proceedings* 1992; 1646: 107-117.
- Lower AM, Coumbe A, Armstrong P, Grudzinskas JG. Initial *in vivo* experience with a new diode laser in gynecological surgery. *Lasers Surg Med* 1994; suppl. 6: 18.
- McHugh JDA. Initial clinical experience using a diode laser in the treatment of retinal vascular disease. *Eye* 1989; 3: 516-527.
- Puliafito CA, Deutsch TF, Boff J, To K. Semiconductor laser endophotocoagulation of the retina. *Arch Ophthalmol* 1987; 105: 424-427.
- Rastegar S, Jacques SL, Motamedi M, Kim BM. Theoretical analysis of equivalency of high-power diode laser (810 nm) and Nd-YAG (1,064 nm) for coagulation of tissue: predictions for prostate coagulation. *SPIE* vol 1646 Laser tissue interaction III, 1992: 150-160.
- Sculpher MJ. A preliminary economic evaluation of the diode laser in ophthalmology. *Lasers Med Sci* 1993; 8: 163-169.
- Watson GM. Use of a semiconductor diode laser in urology. *SPIE* 1993; 1879B: 48.
- Watson GM. Contact laser prostatectomy. *World J Urol* 1995; 13: 115-118.

Index

Aluminium/Gallium Arsenide (Ga Al As) diodes, 41
Anterior base of the skull, 54, 55, 63
Argon, 8, 12, 15, 83
Astrocytomas, 64

Bipolar, 46, 51, 54, 69, 73
Brain stem tumours, 62, 1

Carbon dioxide, 15, 19, 79, 80
Cavernous hemangioma, 62
Cavitron UltraSound Aspiration (CUSA), 9, 44, 54
CO_2 lasers, 8, 9, 13, 19, 21, 22, 64, 81
Coagulation necrosis, 33, 45
Coagulation, 21, 28, 31-34, 43, 45, 54, 65, 69, 80-83
Coherent, 8, 12, 16
Colloid cysts, 48, 64, 79
Contact mode, 28, 42, 43, 46, 47, 49, 51, 54, 56, 59, 61, 62, 65, 67, 69, 70, 72, 73
Craniopharyngiomas, 62

DHE, 75
810 nm diode lasers, 48
Diomed 25/30, 41
Dye lasers, 23

Einstein Albert, 7
Electromagnetic radiation, 7, 14
Electromagnetic spectrum, 11, 12, 27, 41
Emission, 7, 8, 11, 13, 18, 19, 20, 22, 24, 43, 44, 46, 58, 59, 62, 64, 65, 76
Emission power, 17-20, 58, 59, 62
Endoscopes, 64, 65
Endoscopy, 22, 42, 47, 48, 62, 64, 65
Energy pump, 15, 1
Ependymoma, 62, 71, 73, 1
Epilepsy, 67

Erbium (Er-YAG), 22
Eyes, 35, 36

Fibre optic, 9, 21-23, 26, 36, 42, 48, 62, 65
Fluence, 31, 81
Foramen, 55, 60, 63, 65, 66

Generator, 16, 20, 41
Gliomas, 34, 48, 64

Haemostasis, 7, 9, 19, 29, 33, 34, 43, 45, 46, 54, 58, 59, 62, 64, 65, 69, 70, 73
Hand piece, 20, 21, 42, 43, 48, 58, 61
Helium-Neon, 12, 15, 17, 19, 21, 27
Hemangiomas, 73, 1
Holmium (Ho-YAG), 22
HPD (hematoporphyrin), 75
Hyperthermia, 32, 33

Incoherent, 11, 12, 16, 17
Interventional navigation, 26, 46-48, 64, 76
Intracranial tumours, 51
Intramedullary tumours, 67, 72
Intraspinal lipomas, 69
Intraspinal tumours, 67
Intraventricular tumours and colloid cysts, 64
Irradiance, 17, 18, 31

KTP, 22

Laser cavity, 16, 26
Laser fibres, 27, 48, 76
Laser-tissue interactions, 31, 80, 82
LED, 23, 24, 37, 79
Light-emitting diode, 23

Maiman, 8, 81
Maintenance, 37, 38, 42
MASER, 8

Meningiomas of the sphenoid ridge, 54, 55
Meningiomas, 34, 44, 47, 48, 51, 54, 55, 58, 63, 67, 69, 79, 82
Metastases, 47, 64
Micro-neurosurgery, 7
Micromanipulator, 21, 58, 61
Miniaturisation, 23, 75
Monochromatic, 11, 12, 16, 77
Myelotomy, 71, 73

1.06 µm Nd-YAG lasers, 33, 47, 51, 65
1.32 µm Nd-YAG lasers, 33, 49, 65
Nd-YAG, 8, 9, 20, 22, 23, 32, 33, 35, 43, 49, 51, 62, 65, 67, 79-83
Neuroendoscopy, 48
Non-contact mode, 28, 32, 33, 42, 44, 51, 52, 54, 55, 58, 62, 65, 66, 69
Non monochromatic, 11
Non-touch technique, 44

Petro-clival region, 55
Photon, 7, 11, 13-1
Pituitary adenomas, 62
Planck, 7, 11
Planck's constant, 11
Posterior cranial fossa, 9, 44, 54, 55, 58, 59, 63
Power density, 17, 18, 46
Power output, 17, 30, 41, 42, 44, 46, 48, 52, 55, 66, 71

Quantum, 7, 11, 13
Quantum of energy, 13

Regulations, 37, 38
Robotisation, 76

Safety precautions, 35
Sapphires, 28, 29
Schwannomas, 55, 58, 61, 67, 69
Sectioning, 28, 29, 33, 43, 44, 46, 69
Semiconductor diode lasers, 19, 23, 24, 41, 75, 76
Shaped fibres, 28, 29, 42, 46, 58
Skin, 35, 36
Smart lasers, 75
Spatial coherence, 16
Spinal cord, 9, 34, 44, 60, 69, 70
Spontaneous emission, 13, 24
Stereotactic surgery, 46, 47
Stimulated, 7, 8, 11, 14, 15, 24, 81
Supratentorial convexity tumours, 51

Temporal coherence, 16
Tunable pocket lasers, 75

Ultrafast lasers, 76
Unipolar electrocoagulation, 46

Vaporisation, 32, 33, 43, 46, 60, 64, 65
Ventriculocisternostomy, 48, 49, 64, 65, 68
Volatilisation, 44, 76

YAG crystal, 9, 15, 22
YAG lasers, 9, 22, 25